COMPOSING HEALTH LITERACIES

This edited collection examines engagements between health literacies and undergraduate writing instruction, providing research, case studies, and practical guidance on developing an interdisciplinary writing pedagogy.

Bringing together works from scholars in rhetoric and composition, technical communication, UX, public health, nursing, and writing center administration, this collection showcases a range of evidence-based practices for composing, teaching, and assessing health literacies, which the readers can apply to their own contexts. Using non-specialist language accessible to instructors from a variety of backgrounds, the chapters consider the use of writing assignments including image analyses, public service announcements, podcasts, health education materials, illness narratives, public presentations, research proposals, and journal articles. The book offers a holistic overview by profiling entire writing programs, both online and face-to-face, that teach health literacies across their curricula.

This evidence-based collection is essential reading for scholars and instructors in rhetoric and composition, writing in the health professions, technical communication, and health humanities, and can be used as a supplemental textbook for pedagogy courses in these fields.

Michael J. Madson is an Assistant Professor at Arizona State University, USA where he teaches courses in healthcare communication and user experience. He is also an adjunct Associate Professor at the Medical University of South Carolina, USA where he runs an online undergraduate writing course that explores health literacy, bioethics, and interprofessional education. He is the editor of *Teaching writing in the health professions: Perspectives, problems, and practices* (2022).

COMPOSING HEALTH LITERACIES

Perspectives and Resources for Undergraduate Writing Instruction

Edited by Michael J. Madson

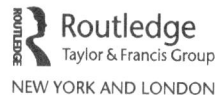

Routledge
Taylor & Francis Group

NEW YORK AND LONDON

Designed cover image: © Getty Images

First published 2023
by Routledge
605 Third Avenue, New York, NY 10158

and by Routledge
4 Park Square, Milton Park, Abingdon, Oxon, OX14 4RN

Routledge is an imprint of the Taylor & Francis Group, an informa business

ISBN: 978-1-032-32798-3 (hbk)
ISBN: 978-1-032-29926-6 (pbk)
ISBN: 978-1-003-31677-0 (ebk)

DOI: 10.4324/9781003316770

Typeset in Bembo
by MPS Limited, Dehradun

To Kent "Duke" Stuetz and Tami Robins, models of fortitude

CONTENTS

CONTRIBUTORS

Elinor Borgert received her Ph.D. in Health Policy and Administration (minoring in Epidemiology) from the University of North Carolina in Chapel Hill. She has served on the faculty at the Medical University of South Carolina in Charleston, SC, USA since 1999, interrupted only by a 5-year term as the Dean of Student Affairs at Belmont University's School of Pharmacy in Nashville, TN, USA.

Elizabeth A. Brown is an academic educator and health services researcher who focuses on social determinants of health, particularly race/ethnicity, access to primary care, health care policy, and chronic conditions. In December 2022, Dr. Brown joined Old Dominion University, USA, where she serves as their Public Health Director for the Bachelor of Science program.

Aaron Bruenger is a Senior Lecturer in the Center for Learning Innovation at the University of Minnesota Rochester, USA. He teaches writing and communication courses in the Bachelor of Science in Health Science and Bachelor of Science in Health Professions programs, and has research interests in pedagogy, rhetorical theory and criticism, narrative theory, and reflective writing/communication.

Karina Daniel is an instructor in the Specialized English Language Programs (SELP) at St. George's University (SGU), Grenada. She is the course director for Communication for the Health Professions I, an academic writing course that focuses on helping pre-medical and pre-veterinary students read, evaluate, and communicate research. This course is the foundation to Communications for the Health Professions II (CHP II), which she taught for three years.

Lauren Geller is the Director of the Division of Healthcare Studies in the Department of Clinical Sciences at the Medical University of South Carolina, USA. Over the past 9 years, Dr. Gellar has led two health professions undergraduate programs which follow a "health literacies across the curriculum" (HLAC) approach. Dr. Gellar has taught the Practicum courses at MUSC for 4 years.

Karen Diane Groller is an Associate Professor for the Helen S. Breidegam School of Nursing and Public Health and is the director of first-year writing at Moravian University, USA. She is a published nurse researcher, educator, and expert in the fields of obesity management, particularly bariatric surgery education practices, and digital education pedagogies.

Michael J. Klein is a Professor of Writing, Rhetoric, and Technical Communication at James Madison University, USA, where he serves as director of the Cohen Center for the Humanities and coordinator of the cross-disciplinary minor in medical humanities. He teaches undergraduate and graduate courses in writing in the health sciences, narrative and graphic medicine, and medical rhetoric, and co-developed a cross-disciplinary course on COVID-19.

Bronson Lemer is a Senior Lecturer in the Center for Learning Innovation at the University of Minnesota Rochester, USA and a 2019 McKnight Writing Fellow.

Michael J. Madson is an Assistant Professor at Arizona State University, USA, where he teaches courses in healthcare communication and user experience. He is also an adjunct Associate Professor at the Medical University of South Carolina, USA, where he runs an online undergraduate writing course that explores health literacy, bioethics, and interprofessional education. He is the editor of *Teaching writing in the health professions: Perspectives, problems, and practices* (2022).

Lucy Bryan Malenke is an Assistant Professor of writing at James Madison University, USA, where she serves as the University Writing Center's liaison to the College of Health and Behavioral Studies. She has created many online resources for writers composing in academic and professional genres in the health professions. Additionally, she provides training to faculty, teaching assistants, and peer tutors on how to best serve such writers.

Katherine E. Morelli currently teaches at Northeastern University, USA, and the University of Massachusetts-Boston, USA. She holds a PhD in Writing, Rhetoric, and Literacies and a MA in Applied Linguistics. In her research, she merges her training and expertise as a linguist and rhetorician to investigate the role of language and culture in health communication and health literacy.

Jill Paterson-Charles is a Language Instructor in the Specialized English Language Programs (SELP) at the St. George's University School of Medicine (SGU), Grenada. As the course director for Communication for the Health Professions II, she has worked with her unit to revamp the course to concentrate more meaningfully on critical thinking within a One Health One Medicine framework and develop writing skills throughout the writing process.

Jarron Slater is currently a Visiting Assistant Professor at Brigham Young University, USA. He previously taught at Valparaiso University, USA, the University of Minnesota – Twin Cities, USA, and Utah Valley University, USA. He studies how the humanities can help people become better professional communicators by providing them with the skills they need to make personal, empathetic, and real connections.

Kirk St.Amant is a Professor and Eunice C. Williamson Endowed Chair in Technical Communication and Research Faculty Member with the Center for Biomedical Engineering and Rehabilitation Science (CBERS) at Louisiana Tech University, USA. He is also an Adjunct Professor of International Health and Medical Communication with the University of Limerick, Ireland, and a Research Fellow and Adjunct Professor of User Experience Design with the University of Strasbourg, France.

Yuko Taniguchi is an Assistant Professor of Medicine and Arts at the Center for Learning Innovation at the University of Minnesota Rochester, USA. Her research and practice focus on designing and delivering creativity-based programs that promote self-exploration, discovery, and awareness through reflective and creative expressions. Her awards include The Dayton Literary Peace Prize, the Kiriyama Prize Notable Book, and the Gustavus Myers Center Outstanding Book Award Advancing Human Rights.

Catherine VanDerwerker is a Research Associate at the Medical University of South Carolina (MUSC), USA. Dr. VanDerwerker's clinical work has focused on inpatient and outpatient neurorehabilitation, especially spinal cord injury and stroke recovery. Now, as a full-time researcher, she is interested in studying the use of exercise and non-invasive brain stimulation in neurological and neuropsychiatric populations to improve depressive symptoms.

Jennifer Wacek is a Senior Lecturer in the Center for Learning Innovation at the University of Minnesota Rochester, USA, where she teaches literature, writing, and capstone courses. She earned her PhD in Comparative Literature at the University of Wisconsin, Madison. Her research interests include the modern novel in English, French, and Arabic, postcolonial literature, literature and gender, and reflective writing pedagogy.

Allison S. Walker is the Director of Service Learning and English instructor at High Point University, USA. Her poems have appeared in numerous literary journals and her research interests include narrative medicine and empathy studies.

Noah Wason is a Lecturer in the Writing Initiative at Binghamton University, USA. His research focuses on the intersections between rhetorical theory and technology, notably the connections between ethos, surveillance, and the algorithmic technologies that power social media platforms. His work has appeared in several publications including *Rhetoric Review*.

Charles Woods is an Assistant Professor at Texas A&M University—Commerce, USA. He studies how society understands digital privacy and his research positions privacy policies as the sites where we can learn about and teach about digital privacy and asymmetrical power. He has won the *Kairos* Service Award, the John Lovas Award, and the *Computers & Composition* Michelle Kendrick Award for producing and hosting "The Big Rhetorical Podcast," which features graduate students and other academics working in rhetoric, writing studies, and technical communication.

INTRODUCTION: THE INTERSECTIONS OF HEALTH LITERACIES AND UNDERGRADUATE WRITING INSTRUCTION

Michael J. Madson

Health literacy, variously defined, is a major concern across borders. National data indicate that in the United States (US), a third of adults had only basic health literacy or below (Kutner et al., 2006). A comparative survey of eight European countries found "insufficient or problematic" levels of health literacy in almost half of the respondents (Sørensen et al., 2015). Few data are available from the developing world, yet the COVID-19 "infodemic" has exposed how health literacy is an underestimated problem globally, exacerbating social and medical disparities (Paakkari & Okan, 2020). The consequences can be serious, both personally and systemtically. Poor health literacy is associated with risky behaviors, ill health, and mismanagement of chronic diseases such as cancer, diabetes, HIV/AIDS, and asthma. Poor health literacy is further associated with higher rates of hospitalization, rehospitalization, and premature death. All this can strain healthcare systems, driving up the costs of care (Kickbusch et al., 2013, p. 7).

The health literacy crisis has inspired action from governmental, clinical, and academic leaders. Recently, Healthy People 2030 adopted an expanded definition of health literacy, one that highlights the roles of not just individuals, but organizations (Santana et al., 2021). Noted scholars Leena Paakkari and Orkan Okan (2020) have similarly stressed that health literacy involves a shared set of practices: it is essential for those seeking information and services, as well as for those who provide them. Educators in the health professions, in nursing particularly, have integrated health literacy into professional curricula (Mosley & Taylor, 2017; Scott, 2016). To date, however, little has been published on the intersections of health literacy and undergraduate writing instruction (UWI), a significant gap.

This introduction makes a case for the book you are now holding in your hands or displaying on your screen. First, it overviews how the concept and

DOI: 10.4324/9781003316770-1

(inter)discipline of health literacy has evolved, driven largely by top-down forces. Second, it reviews UWI scholarship on health literacy, citing salient works from across fields. Third, and finally, it previews the ensuing chapters, which center on a twofold purpose and feature an interdisciplinary cast of contributors.

A Very Short History of Health Literacy

The term "health literacy" emerged in June 1973, when the Will Rogers Conference on Health Education convened in Saranac Lake, New York. There, Scott Simonds, a professor at the University of Michigan, argued that health education was a matter of public trust. He subsequently recommended health literacy standards for schools. In addition, he called on the mass media to encourage good health practices, establish norms for presenting health information, and counter misleading information about health. The healthcare system, too, needed an overhaul, given its prioritization of sick care over illness prevention, including health education (Simonds, 1974).

The term "health literacy" did not immediately catch on, but like Simonds, researchers and policymakers around the globe called for proactive, multi-level approaches to health. These efforts often revolved around an older term, "health promotion," which was coined by the medical historian Henry Sigerist in the 1940s and later popularized by the "Lalonde report" in the 1970s (Lalonde, 1974; Okan, 2019, p. 28). The report proposed a holistic framework for policy development in Canada, and it became recognized as "one of the founding documents in health promotion" (Public Health Agency of Canada, 2001).

In the mid-1980s, Canadian agencies partnered with the World Health Organization to host the first International Conference on Health Promotion, in Ottawa. The conference was "primarily a response to growing expectations for a new public health movement around the world," attracting 200 participants from 36 countries (World Health Organization [WHO], 2022). The historic charter that resulted called for health promotion initiatives in five action areas. According to Okan (2019), a later conference in Jakarta, Indonesia, introduced health literacy as a way to expand the personal skills described in the Ottawa charter (WHO, 1986). These included "health knowledge, self-confidence, self-efficacy, self-empowerment, attitudes, behaviour, future orientation, participation, coping, caring and health sector navigation" (Okan, 2019, p. 28). Around the same time, Australia unveiled new public health goals that connected health skills with education, adapting the WHO "health-promoting schools" strategy (see, e.g., Booth & Samdal, 1997).

An acceleration point came in the mid-aughts when the various drivers of health literacy converged in a powerful way: landmark reports were issued by the Educational Testing Service (Rudd et al., 2004) and the Institute of Medicine (2004); and national surveys on health literacy took place in the United States (Kutner et al., 2006), Canada (Canadian Council on Learning, 2007), and

Australia (Australia Bureau of Statistics, 2006), finding widespread challenges and motivating coordinated responses. Multi-nationally, the Sixth Global Conference on Health Promotion, which convened in Bangkok, Thailand, made health literacy an explicit focus. Health literacy was considered an important element of state capacity building (see Catford, 2005).

Since then, publications on health literacy have surged. Analyzing the Web of Science database, Qi et al. (2021) found that there were more than 100 publications that addressed health literacy in the year 2009. By 2019, that number crested 9,000. This health literacy scholarship came from about 1,800 authors in 80 countries – especially the United States, the United Kingdom, and Australia – and was published in more than 1,600 journals. Most of these journals are devoted to medicine and public health. Health literacy scholarship has also expanded into the fields of education, psychology, and other social sciences, and currently, health literacy research appears to be following four streams: how health literacy relates to specific illnesses and conditions, patient populations, various means of receiving information, and scholarship in languages other than English. Of note, little work on health literacy has come from South America, South Asia, the Arab states, Russia, and the Slavic countries in Europe (Qi et al., 2021).

Few studies to date have focused specifically on what health literacy means, but the definitions are numerous, raising challenges for scholarship and instruction. It appears that the first systematic review in this area was done by Sørensen et al. (2012), who identified 12 models and 17 definitions. Four years later, Malloy-Weir et al. (2016) identified 250 definitions (!). Amid this conceptual diversity, however, three definitions have been particularly influential.

One is from the American Medical Association (1999): health literacy is a "constellation of skills, including the ability to perform basic reading and numerical tasks required to function in the health care environment," including the "ability to read and comprehend prescription bottles, appointment slips, and other essential health-related materials."

Another is associated with the Institute of Medicine: the "degree to which individuals have the capacity to obtain, process, and understand basic health information and services needed to make appropriate health decisions" (Ratzan & Parker, 2000). This definition circulated widely with the influential publication *Health literacy: A prescription to end confusion* (Nielsen-Bohlman et al., 2004).

Another definition was developed by the World Health Organization (1998): "cognitive and social skills which determine the motivation and ability of individuals to gain access to, understand and use information in ways which promote and maintain good health."

These three definitions, though generative, have been limited somewhat by their emphasis on individual, functional literacies. Recognizing this limitation, recent scholarship has situated health literacy in the wider orbits of culture, context, and language. Don Nutbeam (2000), for example, has described two additional types of health literacy: interactive and critical. Interactive health literacy is competencies needed for daily living, including the ability to apply new information amid changing circumstances. Critical health literacy refers to the capacity to evaluate health information, use it, and exert greater control over life events. Nutbeam (2000) maintains that students can (and should) acquire these literacies through formal education, in addition to out-of-class personal experiences.

Within these wider orbits, health literacy is more than a clinical risk or individual asset. Health literacy is tangled up in issues of transparency, access, and rights. It is a powerful mediator of social determinants of health, and even a form of health citizenship (Kickbusch, 2004). Subsequently, scholars have called greater attention to the roles that organizations play. Like health literacy in general, organizational health literacy is a heterogenous concept that spans theories and operational frameworks, and studies have illuminated its connections to population health, public health, responsive practice, and cultural competence (Farmanova et al., 2018).

Forms of organizational health literacy have been recognized by the Australian Commission on Quality and Safety in Healthcare (2013), as well as the Organisation for Economic Cooperation and Development (Moreira, 2018). More recently, it was also recognized by the Healthy People 2030 program, which adopted a twofold definition, personal and organizational:

> *Personal health literacy* is the degree to which individuals have the ability to find, understand, and use information and services to inform health related decisions and actions for themselves and others.
>
> *Organizational health literacy* is the degree to which organizations equitably enable individuals to find, understand, and use information and services to inform health-related decisions and actions for themselves and others.

The twofold definition arose from lengthy discussion among working groups as well as 187 public comments that were analyzed both internally and externally (Santana et al., 2021, p. S261). It has several significant differences from the Ratzan and Parker (2000) definition used in prior Healthy People programs. First, the definition of personal health literacy emphasizes the *use* of health information and services, shifts from *appropriate decisions* to *informed decisions and actions*, and includes a public health perspective that promotes the health of self and others. Second, the definition of organizational health literacy emphasizes that health literacy is contextual and that organizations must address health literacy in equitable ways. The hope is that the twofold definition will spark improvements in patients' understanding of health information, patient/provider communication, and shared decision-making.

Around the world, there have been additional developments. For example, Canada, Australia, China, the United Kingdom, and Finland have made health literacy a national strategy. Building on the European Health Literacy Project, which took place from 2009 to 2012, the European Health Literacy Conference has been held regularly since 2011 (Health Literacy Europe, 2020). The WHO Southeast Asia Region has introduced a health literacy toolkit for low- and middle-income countries, which is intended to help communities generate their own solutions (Dodson et al., 2015). Moreover, the United Nations Economic and Social Council (2009) has issued this bold declaration: "We stress that health literacy is an important factor in ensuring significant health outcomes, and in this regard, call for the development of appropriate action plans to promote health literacy." In support, the ninth Global Conference on Health Promotion, held in Shanghai, made health literacy one of its three thematic pillars, along with healthy cities and good governance (World Health Organization, 2017).

This very short history suggests how health literacy, as a concept and (inter) discipline, has developed rapidly over the past two decades. It seems clear that more voices across more geographies are needed, and that the teaching of health literacy is of paramount importance, as Scott Simonds (1974) initially argued at Saranac Lake. The "education for health literacy" movement has picked up more steam in recent years, appealing to scholars and teachers across fields (Vamos et al., 2020). But in these efforts, UWI has played only a peripheral role.

Health Literacy in/and UWI

UWI is a vast area of research and pedagogical practice that is largely, but not exclusively, parceled among composition pedagogy, technical communication, rhetorical studies, community literacy, and related fields. We believe that UWI can do much to promote health literacy, and for several reasons.

One reason is the number of students that UWI impacts worldwide. In the United States, the National Census on Writing (2017) found that 97% of the responding two- ($n = 40$) and four-year ($n = 410$) institutions had writing requirements. Universities in South America, notably Colombia, have an institutional policy to offer one or two freshman composition courses (Cardona, 2019; see also Bazerman et al., 2017). Similarly, in the European Higher Education Area, it is common to assess undergraduate learning through writing (European Commission, n.d.). In the Gulf Cooperation Countries, writing requirements have proliferated in recent years, partly due to the establishment of international branch campuses (Rudd & Relafici, 2017). Thus, undergraduate writing instructors are a sizeable force, including in countries where health literacy scholarship and policies are lacking where health literacy scholarship and policies are lacking.

Another reason is the theoretical and methodological vitality of UWI. UWI teacher-scholars have produced hundreds of works related to health and medicine generally –monographs, edited collections, journal special issues, and international conference presentations.[1] The UWI literature specific to health literacy has been more modest, with growing streams on assignments and course designs. For instance, Ward (2021) designed activities and assessments around ethnocultural empathy: the ability to perceive the world through the eyes of a racial or ethnic Other. Forsa (2018) described a "writing about health" course that foregrounded rhetorical decision-making. Students presented about health in the news, analyzed a academic journal article and patient education brochure, produced a brochure themselves, and wrote a grant. Kenzie and McCall (2018) created a course that integrates the medical humanities, the rhetoric of health and medicine, and disability studies. Rose et al. (2008) examined a novel pedagogy, "scaffolding academic literacy," to support indigenous students in the health sciences, drawing on systemic functional linguistics.

If expanded, these streams may provide deeper insight into the ethical premises of teaching health literacy (the "why"), the content of health literacy instruction (the "what"), and the tone of health literacy instruction (the "how") (Paakkari & George, 2018). These streams may inform the health professions, in particular. According to a systematic review by Saunders et al. (2019), few health literacy education interventions have emphasized writing, and these have been functional in focus. As an illustration, some students in the health professions were tasked to rewrite medication information in plain language or, using a readability instrument, assess patient education materials (Saunders et al., 2019). More robust interventions, within the health sciences and in other majors, could apply principles of "writing to learn" (van Dijk et al., 2022). There is a parallel need to establish more longitudinal, programmatic approaches, cultivating health literacy beyond a single assignment or course.

UWI scholarship has also started to engage critically and directly with the meaning of health literacy. Notably, Opel (2018) critiqued the ways that government programs in the United States present the Health Literate Care model. According to Opel (2018), the model does have some benefits, such as highlighting the roles of the healthcare system in supporting patient health literacy. Yet, the system's fragmentation and brokenness can be masked by claims about low health literacy in the community. Lee and Hickman (2018) likewise critiqued dominant models of health literacy in clinical contexts. These authors explained that, across definitions, health literacy has been understood as "a skills-based process used to identify and transform information into knowledge" (p. 76). They subsequently argued for greater complexity, considering power relations, histories, and the resources that patients bring to clinic, such as personal values, emotions, and prior knowledge. In their view, such complexity can be better captured by the plural term "health literacies," as opposed to the singular "health literacy."

A third reason is an ethical and professional imperative. As Melonçon and Frost (2015) wrote nearly a decade ago:

> Scholars in communication, technical and professional communication, and rhetoric and composition have recognized that we have the potential to play increasingly important roles on interdisciplinary health research teams, to help improve patient-centered language and practices across a multitude of media and document types, and to contribute to solving such problems as the health literacy crisis that leaves some 90 million Americans unable to process the most basic health information. (p. 7)

This crisis continues to impact institutions of higher education, where many undergraduates have limited health literacy themselves (Juvinyà-Canal, 2020; Patil et al., 2021; Rababah et al., 2019). Yet, we believe that writing classrooms, physical or digital, may be ideal spaces for interventions, and undergraduate writing instructors can be a significant force in the "education for health literacy" movement (see Vamos et al., 2020). In turn, health literacy topics can enrich UWI assignments, courses, and programs, and health literacy scholarship in other fields can enhance studies in UWI. In short, the intersections between health literacy and UWI, though underexplored, have strong potential to be mutually beneficial.

Purpose, Organization, and Key Features of the Collection

Responding to the exigencies above, *Composing health literacies* has a twofold purpose:

- To dig into the intersection of UWI and health literacies conceptually, encouraging additional scholarship; and
- To illustrate evidence-based practices for teaching and assessing health literacies, which UWI instructors can apply to their own contexts.

Following this introduction, the 11 body chapters are organized into three parts.

Part I: Assignments and courses. The five chapters in this part spotlight undergraduate writing assignments and courses that the contributors have implemented successfully: Karen Diane Groller, a nursing professor, shares her experience teaching health literacies in a first-year writing class, where she incorporates process pedagogy and multimodal design (Chapter 1). Kasey Larson and colleagues, who teach at a university in the West Indies, explain the importance of critical thinking. As an illustration, they analyze a lengthy proposal paper that they assign to students who are actively preparing for medical or veterinary school (Chapter 2). Allison S. Walker links health literacies with empathy, overviewing humanistic classroom activities that have proven effective (Chapter 3).

Jarron Slater picks up on that discussion, demonstrating how "rhetorical aesthetics" can enhance reflection (Chapter 4). To conclude this part of the collection, Michael J. Klein discusses vaccine health literacies, sharing insights from his students' work with community agencies in Virginia (Chapter 5).

Part II: Programs. The four chapters in this part profile programs, online or face to face, that make extensive use of health literacies: Lucy Bryan Malenke furnishes tools for exploring a kind of organizational health literacies; in particular, she reports on an initiative to develop and assess knowledge, skills, and attitudes for writing in a Health Sciences major (Chapter 6). Yuko Taniguchi and colleagues explain the four-year assignment sequence used at their institution, a campus of fewer than 1,000 undergraduates, to cultivate reflective practice (Chapter 7). Rounding out this part, my colleagues and I describe an online program developed at an academic health sciences center, which deploys an approach that we call "health literacies across the curriculum" (Chapter 8).

Part III: Extensions. The three chapters here detail theoretical work and field studies that can inform classroom instruction, extending the boundaries of health literacies and UWI: Katherine E.Morelli distills instructional implications from her research on cultural health navigators, who worked at a refugee clinic in the US. Southwest (Chapter 9). The cultural health navigators hail from Somalia, Burundi, Burma, and Iraq. Charles Woods and Noah Wason parse the intricacies of health information collected by wearable technologies, and they take Apple Watch policies as an illustrative case, highlighting data usage, transparency, and privacy (Chapter 10). Finally, Kirk St.Amant connects health literacies with prototype theory, which can inform usability tests in health and medical contexts (Chapter 11).

The chapters thus provide a "dialogue across differing epistemological positions" (Opel, 2018, p. 44), capturing a broad spectrum of UWI settings, tasks, and supporting topics. Indeed, the contributors discuss first-year writing, advanced composition, technical communication, writing program administration, and the health sciences. They describe public service announcements (some in the form of infographics and podcasts), proposals, reflections, parallel charts, poems, pathographies, patient education materials, article critiques, "unessays," research reports, formal presentations, prototyped content, and more. Alongside the central focus on health literacies, the contributors explore multimodality and digital literacy, critical thinking, problem-based learning, the health humanities, empathy, narrative medicine, aesthetics, vaccine education, service learning, deliberate practice, interprofessional education, reflective practice, collaborative research, mental models, and intercultural knowledge – topics that can energize UWI, no matter the students' majors.

Acknowledging the breadth of UWI, the chapters were composed with two primary audiences in mind. One is instructors of undergraduate students considering health-related careers, such as majors in pre-med, pre-veterinary, dental assisting, health sciences, nursing, or surgical technology. Research has shown that writing instruction is instrumental for students' acquisition of academic health literacies, workplace health literacies, as well as personal qualities, including empathy and reflection, that will be key in their future work (see Madson, 2022). Furthermore, these students may be entering health literacy environments where dis/misinformation is increasingly common, they may serve patients with low levels of health literacy, and they may deliver services over both physical and digital modalities. As emphasized in Shanghai declaration, "Engaging health promotion leaders of tomorrow" is critical (WHO, p. 19).

The other is instructors who teach undergraduate students entering careers outside of healthcare, but who wish to integrate health literacies into their courses and programs. As a mode of inquiry, writing instruction can help students, no matter their majors or career paths, cultivate a diversity of health literacies, including critical thought about the healthcare systems serving their communities. These are important competencies, enabling students to "get a better understanding of their health options and take more control over their health decisions" (Moreira, 2018, p. 10).

All of the contributors engage with the idea of health literacies, either head-on or at an angle. Yet, while reading, you may notice that we do not offer definitive resolutions to the challenges of conceptualizing and teaching health literacies. We may even offer as many knots as unknottings. Clearly, there is much more work to be done on health literacies and UWI, and our hope is that this collection will prompt more exploration. Ultimately, that exploration may further nuance assessment discourses, moving beyond polarities of "high" and "low." That exploration may foster greater equity and social justice, given the relationships between health literacies and social determinants of health. Eventually, that exploration may nudge cities, countries, and regions closer to the Sustainable Development Goals (United Nations Development Programme, 2022) and towards a Health in All Policies strategy (see Centers for Disease Control and Prevention, 2016). In the end, although we diverge in many ways, all of the contributors agree without reservation that health literacies "can't be ignored" (Moreira, 2018, p.11), and we invite you to join with us as a scholar, teacher, and advocate.

Note

1 As a "pulse check," I searched the CompPile database, which has cataloged more than 113,000 citations in 303 indexed journals. Currently, the database shows 211 records that contain the keyword "medicine," and another 412 that contain "health," a not insignificant number.

References

American Medical Association, Ad Hoc Committee on health literacy for the Council on Academic Affairs. (1999). Health literacy: Report of the council on academic affairs. *JAMA*, 281(16), 552–557.

Australian Bureau of Statistics (2006). Adult Literacy and Life Skills Survey, Summary Results, Australia, 2006. ABS, Canberra, Catalogue No. 4228.0. www.abs.gov.au

Australian Commission on Safety and Quality in Health Care. (2013). *Consumers, the health system and health literacy: Taking action to improve safety and quality.* Consultation Paper. Sydney, NSW: ACSQHC.

Bazerman, C., Bork, A. V., Poliseli Corrêa, F., Cristovão, V. L., Tapia Ladino, M., Narváez Cardona, E., & Ávila Reyes, N. (2017). Intellectual orientations of studies of higher education writing in Latin America. In S. Plane, C. Bazerman, F. Rondelli, C. Donahue, A. N. Applebee, C. Boré, P. Carlino, M. M. Larruy, P. Rogers, & D. R. Russell (Eds.), *Research on writing: Multiple perspectives* (pp. 281–297). WAC Clearinghouse.

Booth, M. L., & Samdal, O. (1997). Health-promoting schools in Australia: Models and measurement. *Australian and New Zealand Journal of Public Health*, 21(4), 365–370.

Canadian Council on Learning. (2007). *Health literacy in Canada: Initial results from the International Adult Literacy and Skills Survey 2007.* Ottawa: Canadian Council on Learning.

Cardona, E. N. (2019). Writing expectations in a Colombian major in industrial engineering (pp. 371–392). In C. Bazerman, B. Y. G. Pinzón, D. Russell, P. Rogers, L. B., Peña, E. Narváez, P. Carlino, M. Castelló, & M. Tapia-Ladino, (Eds.), *Conocer la escritura: Investigación más allá de las frontera | Knowing writing: Writing research across borders* (pp. 371–392). WAC Clearinghouse.

Catford, J. (2005). The Bangkok Conference: Steering countries to build national capacity for health promotion. *Health Promotion International*, 20, 1–6.

Centers for Disease Control and Prevention. (2016, June 9). *Health in all policies.* Office of the Associate Director for Policy and Strategy. https://www.cdc.gov/policy/hiap/index.html

Dodson, S., Good, S., & Osborne, R. H. (2015). *Health literacy toolkit for low and middle-income countries: A series of information sheets to empower communities and strengthen health systems.* New Delhi: World Health Organization, Regional Office for South-East Asia. Available at: https://apps.who.int/iris/bitstream/handle/10665/205244/B5148.pdf?sequence=1&isAllowed=y

European Commission. (n.d.). *Higher education in Europe.* European Education Area. https://education.ec.europa.eu/study-in-europe/planning-your-studies/higher-education-in-europe

Farmanova, E., Bonneville, L., & Bouchard, L. (2018). Organizational health literacy: Review of theories, frameworks, guides, and implementation issues. *INQUIRY: The Journal of Health Care Organization, Provision, and Financing*, 55, 1–17.

Forsa, C. Q. (2018). Writing about health: A health writing course that emphasizes rhetorical flexibility and teaches for transfer. *Double Helix*, 6, 1–21.

Health Literacy Europe. (2020). The history: Looking back. https://www.healthliteracyeurope.net/history.

Institute of Medicine. (2004). *Health literacy: A prescription to end confusion.* Washington, DC: National Academies Press.

Juvinyà-Canal, D., Suñer-Soler, R., Boixadós Porquet, A., Vernay, M., Blanchard, H., & Bertran-Noguer, C. (2020). Health literacy among health and social care university students. *International Journal of Environmental Research and Public Health*, 17(7), 2273.

Kenzie, D., & McCall, M. (2018). Teaching writing for the health professions: Disciplinary intersections and pedagogical practice. *Technical Communication Quarterly*, 27(1), 64–79.

Kickbusch, I. (2004, October). Improving health literacy – A key priority for enabling good health in Europe. Background paper for the Special Interest Session, European Health Forum, Gastein.

Kickbusch, I., Pelikan, J. M., Apfel, F., & Tsouros, A. D. (Eds.). (2013). *Health literacy: The solid facts.* Copenhagen, Denmark: World Health Organization Regional Office for Europe.

Kutner, M., Greenburg, E., Jin, Y., & Paulsen, C. (2006). The health literacy of America's adults: Results from the 2003 National Assessment of Adult Literacy. NCES 2006-483. *National Center for Education Statistics.*

Lalonde, M. (1974). *A new perspective on the health of Canadians. A working document (Lalonde report).* Ottawa, ON: Government of Canada.

Lee, J. N., & Hickman, A. C. (2018). Keyword essay: Health literacy. *Community Literacy Journal*, 12(2), 73–83.

Madson, M. J. (Ed.). (2022). *Teaching writing in the health professions: Perspectives, problems, and practices.* Routledge.

Malloy-Weir, L. J., Charles, C., Gafni, A., & Entwistle, V. (2016). A review of health literacy: Definitions, interpretations, and implications for policy initiatives. *Journal of Public Health Policy*, 37(3), 334–352.

Melonçon, L., & Frost, E. A. (2015). Special issue introduction: Charting an emerging field: The rhetorics of health and medicine and its importance in communication design. *Communication Design Quarterly Review*, 3(4), 7–14.

Moreira, L. (2018). *Health literacy for people-centred care: Where do OECD countries stand?* Paris, France: Organisation for Economic Cooperation and Development. 10.1787/d8494d3a-en

Mosley, C. M., & Taylor, B. J. (2017). Integration of health literacy content into nursing curriculum utilizing the health literacy expanded model. *Teaching and Learning in Nursing*, 12(2), 109–116.

National Census on Writing. (2017). *Two-year institution survey and Four-year institution survey.* Available at https://writingcensus.ucsd.edu/

Nielsen-Bohlman, L., Panzer, A. M., & Kindig, D. A. (2004). *Health literacy: A prescription to end confusion.* Washington, D.C.: The National Academies Press.

Nutbeam, D. (2000). Health literacy as a public health goal: A challenge for contemporary health education and communication strategies into the 21st century. *Health Promotion International*, 15(3), 259–267.

Office of Disease Prevention and Health Promotion. (n.d.). *Health literacy in Healthy People 2030.* Healthy People 2030. https://health.gov/healthypeople/priority-areas/health-literacy-healthy-people-2030

Okan, O. (2019). From Saranac Lake to Shanghai: A brief history of health literacy. In O. Okan, U. Bauer, D. Levin-Zamir, P. Pinheiro, & K. Sørensen (Eds.), *International handbook of health literacy: Research, practice and policy across the lifespan* (pp. 21–37). Policy Press.

Opel, D. S. (2018). Challenging the rhetorical conception of health literacy: Aging, interdependence, and networked caregiving. *Literacy in Composition Studies*, 6(2), 136–150.

Paakkari, L., & George, S. (2018). Ethical underpinnings for the development of health literacy in schools: Ethical premises ('why'), orientations ('what') and tone ('how'). *BMC Public Health*, 18(1), 1–10.

Paakkari, L., & Okan, O. (2020). COVID-19: Health literacy is an underestimated problem. *The Lancet Public Health*, 5(5), e249–e250.

Patil, U., Kostareva, U., Hadley, M., Manganello, J. A., Okan, O., Dadaczynski, K., ... & Sentell, T. (2021). Health literacy, digital health literacy, and COVID-19 pandemic attitudes and behaviors in US college students: Implications for interventions. *International Journal of Environmental Research and Public Health*, 18(6), 3301.

Public Health Agency of Canada. (2001, December 8). *A new perspective on the health of Canadians*. Government of Canada. https://www.canada.ca/en/public-health/services/health-promotion/population-health/a-new-perspective-on-health-canadians.html

Qi, S., Hua, F., Xu, S., Zhou, Z., & Liu, F. (2021). Trends of global health literacy research (1995–2020): Analysis of mapping knowledge domains based on citation data mining. *Plos One*, 16(8), e0254988.

Rababah, J. A., Al-Hammouri, M. M., Drew, B. L., & Aldalaykeh, M. (2019). Health literacy: Exploring disparities among college students. *BMC Public Health*, 19(1), 1–11.

Ratzan, S. C., & Parker, R. M. (2000). Introduction. In C. R. Selden, M. Zorn, & R. M. Ratzan (eds.), *National Library of Medicine Current Bibliographies in Medicine: Health Literacy, NLM Pub. No. CMB 2000-1* (pp. v–vi). Bethesda, MD: National Institutes of Health, U.S. Department of Health and Human Services.

Rose, D., Rose, M., Farrington, S., & Page, S. (2008). Scaffolding academic literacy with indigenous health sciences students: An evaluative study. *Journal of English for Academic Purposes*, 7(3), 165–179.

Rudd, M., & Relafici, M. (2017). An Arabian gulf: First-year composition textbooks at an international branch campus in Qatar. In L. R. Arnold, A. Nebel, & L. Ronesi, (Eds.), *Emerging writing research from the Middle East-North Africa region* (pp. 115–132). WAC Clearinghouse.

Rudd, R., Kirsch, I., & Yamamoto, K. (2004). *Literacy and health in America*. Policy Information Report. Princeton, NJ: Educational Testing Service.

Santana, S., Brach, C., Harris, L., Ochiai, E., Blakey, C., Bevington, F., ... & Pronk, N. (2021). Practice Full Report: Updating health literacy for Healthy People 2030: Defining Its importance for a new decade in public health. *Journal of Public Health Management and Practice*, 27(6 Supp.), S258–S264. doi: 10.1097/PHH.0000000000001324

Saunders, C., Palesy, D., & Lewis, J. (2019). Systematic review and conceptual framework for health literacy training in health professions education. *Health Professions Education*, 5(1), 13–29.

Scott, S. A. (2016). Health literacy education in baccalaureate nursing programs in the United States. *Nursing Education Perspectives*, 37(3), 153–158.

Simonds, S. K. (1974). Health education as social policy. *Health Education Monograph*, 2, 1–25.

Sørensen, K., Pelikan, J. M., Röthlin, F., Ganahl, K., Slonska, Z., Doyle, G., ... & Brand, H. (2015). Health literacy in Europe: Comparative results of the European health literacy survey (HLS-EU). *European Journal of Public Health*, 25(6), 1053–1058.

Sørensen, K., Van den Broucke, S., Fullam, J., Doyle, G., Pelikan, J., Slonska, Z., & Brand, H. (2012). Health literacy and public health: A systematic review and integration of definitions and models. *BMC Public Health*, 12(1), 1–13.

United Nations Development Programme. (2022). *Sustainable Development Goals*. https://www.undp.org/sustainable-development-goals

United Nations Economic and Social Council. (2009). Ministerial Declaration – 2009 High level segment: Implementing the internationally agreed goals and commitments in regard to global public health. Available at: https://www.un.org/en/ecosoc/newfunct/amrdocumentation2009.shtml

Vamos, S., Okan, O., Sentell, T., & Rootman, I. (2020). Making a case for "Education for health literacy": An international perspective. *International Journal of Environmental Research and Public Health*, 17(4), 1436.

van Dijk, A., van Gelderen, A., & Kuiken, F. (2022). Which types of instruction in writing-to-learn lead to insight and topic knowledge in different disciplines? A review of empirical studies. *Review of Education*, 10(2), e3359.

Van Rensburg, J. Z. (2020). Levels of health literacy and English comprehension in patients presenting to South African primary healthcare facilities. *African Journal of Primary Health Care and Family Medicine*, 12(1), 1–6.

Ward, M. (2021). Embedding ethnocultural empathy in a community-based health intervention writing assignment. *Prompt: A Journal of Academic Writing Assignments*, 5(1), 54–62.

World Health Organization. (1986). *The Ottawa Charter for health promotion: First international conference on health promotion*, Ottawa, 21 November, Geneva: WHO.

World Health Organization. (1998). Health promotion glossary. http://www.who.int/healthpromotion/about/HPG/en/

World Health Organization. (2017). Shanghai Declaration on promoting health in the 2030 Agenda for Sustainable Development. *Health Promotion International*, 32(1), 7–8.

World Health Organization. (2022). *Health promotion: Overview*. https://www.who.int/health-topics/health-promotion#tab=tab_1

PART I
Assignments and Courses

1

ENGAGING HEALTH LITERACIES THROUGH MULTIMODAL PROJECTS IN FIRST-YEAR WRITING

Karen Diane Groller

On a daily basis, more than half of the world's population engages with "new" media, such as blogs, wiki, memes, podcasts, and infographics (DataReportal, 2021a; DataReportal, 2021b; Pew Research Center, 2021). Young adults often use new media to attain health information. The National Institutes of Health, noticing similar behavior in older adults, has created educational guides on how to consume online health information critically (National Institute on Aging, 2022). Other organizations, such as the World Health Organization (WHO) and the Centers for Disease Control and Prevention (CDC), have also become active in new media. These digital practices require a kind of health literacies that support development of both analytical consumers and accountable producers of health information, which is why colleges and universities should consider incorporating this topic in undergraduate writing instruction (Groller, 2018).

Writing activities can actively engage learners, including future health professionals, in analyzing and producing public messages related to health. A designated course such as first-year writing (FYW) may be ideal because it offers ample time to learn about writing while exploring health literacies as a concept and set good writing practices. Furthermore, FYW can encourage connections to learners' intended health disciplines, provide a structured setting for investigating new media, and consider how new media may influence individual and community health. This chapter shares the guiding framework and assignment sequences that I have used to teach health literacies in such a setting, providing resources for other instructors.

Guiding Framework

To guide my teaching as a FYW instructor and nurse educator, I draw on Anne Beaufort's (2007) five knowledge domains. I blend these domains with theories

DOI: 10.4324/9781003316770-3

of multimodality, including digital genres. While all writing is multimodal, I found these theories particularly helpful when working with new media, supporting learner project designs. So can knowledge of information, digital, and rhetorical literacies and principles of teaching for transfer. Below, I provide a quick summary of these areas.

Beaufort's (2007) Five Knowledge Domains

Beaufort (2007) described five knowledge domains that can facilitate undergraduate writing instruction: process, genre, subject matter, discourse community, and rhetorical knowledge. Briefly, the writing process moves from conceptualization to revision and potentially publication. Genre refers to how knowledge is communicated through traditional and new media forms (more on this below). Subject matter knowledge requires the writer to have knowledge in a particular field and critical thinking to form new information. A discourse community is defined as a group engaged in communication, and the members can serve as contributors, participants, or both. In essence, the discourse community comprises the audiences that learners are writing for, along with their collaborators. Last, rhetorical knowledge enables writers to effectively and efficiently communicate in a way fitting a particular situation (Beaufort, 2007).

Multimodality

Multimodality essentially means "more than just text," and Ball et al. (2022) explain how linguistic, visual, aural, gestural, and spatial modes can all be involved in messaging (see also Ball & Charlton, 2015; Cope & Kalantzis, 2009; Fodrey et al., 2019). The basic meaning of these modes, along with design elements that we have discussed in my FYW courses, are shown in Table 1.1.

TABLE 1.1 Five modes of communication, their basic meanings, and design elements that we have discussed in my FYW writing courses

Mode	Its basic meaning	Design elements
Linguistic	Written or spoken language	Words or numbers that accompany other visual elements
Visual	Cues of various kinds that can be seen	Color, layout, style, size, perspective, and placement (or framing) of objects and text
Aural	Sound	Voices or music, including the use of silence or white noise, tone, emphasis and accents, and volume
Gestural	Body language	Facial expressions, hand gestures, body language, and observed interactions
Spatial	The proximity or distance between design elements	The physical arrangement of objects or people

Digital Genres

To classify digital genres, scholars have applied Swales's (1990) model, which consists of purpose, structure, and intended rhetorical situation (Askehave & Nielsen, 2005). According to Askehave and Nielsen (2005), digital genre theory expands the Swalesian model by recognizing the challenge of categorizing new media forms, which can be richly multimodal.

In some understandings of this theory, digital genres can be determined by the primary form and function of the final products. These may be website layouts, blog entries, vlog live streams, podcast episodes, infographics, memes, advertisements, public service announcements, electronic books and games, and more (Bronstein, 2017; Guslyakova et al., 2018; Rattan, 2019). For each new media genre, there are potentially limitless subgenres, or "subspecies," due to ongoing innovation and information exchange. Take TikTok videos as an example. TikTok is a social media platform that allows users to upload brief videos. Within the platform's creative constraints, common subspecies of TikTok videos currently include challenge dances, lip-synch routines, product promotions, pranks, stunts, and tutorials (Bailey, 2020). These subspecies can be divided into even smaller categories and can blend together. A "what I eat in a day" video, to provide just one illustration, may promote the use of particular food products while teaching viewers how to cook new recipes. Communication attributes of these videos may influence consumers to believe creation and consumption of posted recipes are ideal (or not) for their health.

Take memes, visual forms in new media, as another example. Memes can easily spread from person to person and generate amusement or interest (Groller, 2018). A meme displayed as a captioned static picture or video sets the rhetorical situation in a manner that elicits sarcasm or humor to the discourse community. Memes exhibiting humor or sarcasm around health concepts can impact beliefs and behaviors (Groller, 2018). The result may influence health, especially if the discourse community misinterprets the intended humor or sarcasm from the meme or considers false information to be true. For example, in the recent coronavirus (COVID-19) pandemic, many memes about vaccines and facemasks were shared online that contained false or outdated information, which likely contributed to an increase of doubt, fear, anxiety, and resistance to public health efforts.

These subspecies will continue to evolve as the needs, interests, and preferences of the participants change or as the media company itself alters what is technologically possible.

Information, Digital, and Rhetorical Literacies

To be health literate, undergraduates should acquire information literacies, digital literacies, and rhetorical literacies. According to the American Library

Association (1989), information literacy is the "ability to recognize when information is needed" as well as "the ability to locate, evaluate, and use effectively the needed information" (para. 3). Nurse educators recognize the importance of information literacy, which has been applied in undergraduate BSN programs (Groller et al., 2020).

Simply defined, digital literacy is "the ability to find, evaluate, utilize, share and create content using information technologies and the internet" (Lynch, 2017; para. 2). Fodrey and colleagues (2019) expanded on the definition as "the ability to understand and use technological tools in order to find and critically read audio, visual, spatial, gestural, and/or alphanumeric texts in digital spaces and/or create audio, visual, spatial, gestural, and/or alphanumeric text appropriate for specific digital spaces (Appendix 1)."

Across media, physical or digital, rhetorical literacy leads learners to engage, synthesize and reflect. This form of literacy occurs through "(1) immersion in print culture and appreciation for literary reading, (2) respect for the slowness or 'timelessness' required for deep reflection, (3) practice using rhetorical methods and analyzing discourse though a variety of lenses (contextualizing), and (4) metacognition" (Fodrey et al., 2019, Appendix 1; Schnarr, 2018).

These three literacies come together in multimodal writing projects. As described in *Writer/Designer*, educators should carefully scaffold digital multimodal writing projects from conceptualization to digital dissemination and maintenance (Ball et al., 2022). Such projects enable learners to fuse together informational and digital literacies knowledge as they create a useable product (Bradshaw & Porter, 2017; Chicca & Chunta, 2020; Groller, 2018, Groller et al., 2020). In Chapter 10, Charles Woods and Noah Wason dive deeper into some of these literacies.

Teaching for Transfer

FYW instructors should explicitly teach for transfer. That is, we should frame writing tasks with general concepts so learners can better apply what they have learned to new situations. Using terms such as discourse community, genre, subject matter, and rhetorical situation can help (Beaufort, 2012).

Teaching for transfer can be illustrated by a research paper that requires learners to apply strategies from similar assignments, but to discuss a new topic for a different audience and purpose. With multimodality, teaching for transfer can center on new media, prompting learners to practice foundational writing concepts along with design principles that can apply across modes. Educators integrating health literacies into their undergraduate writing classrooms might ask learners to design health messages, such as public service announcements (PSA) through infographics or podcasts, which we have done at Moravian University.

Institutional Context

Moravian University, located in Bethlehem, Pennsylvania blends liberal arts with professional undergraduate and graduate programs. Moravian University has provided unified access to teaching and learning by equipping both faculty and learners with three devices; a MacBook, iPad, and Apple Pencil, since 2014 (Cantens, 2020). Due to the institution's commitment to innovating education for the 21st century, Moravian College (which became a university in May 2021) became an Apple Distinguished School® in 2018 (Corr, 2019b) and in 2019 accepted an invitation to join the New American Colleges and Universities consortium (Cantens, 2020; Corr, 2019a). The New American Colleges and Universities (2020) consortium consists of small to midsize higher education institutions which demonstrate the integration of the liberal arts, with professional preparation, and civic engagement in a meaningful way.

Moravian's commitment to meaningful and practical learning experiences, along with the established Writing at Moravian (WAM) program, has created a strong writing-enriched curriculum (WEC) culture. In 2022, the program received the Conference on College Composition and Communication Writing Program Certificate of Excellence Award from the National Council of Teachers of English. Consisting of three phases, WEC is a WAM initiative that nurtures connections between learners' writing abilities and discipline-specific practices, preparing learners for their future careers. In terms of sequence, learners start with FYW course, which introduces key concepts related to writing and multimodal design. Transfer is encouraged through additional, writing-intensive courses in the learners' majors, health related or not, and faculty take ownership of writing instruction and assessment (Fodrey & Hassay, 2021).

The FYW course-specific objectives are intended to empower learners to be analytical consumers and accountable producers of digital health messages conveyed in new media. Learners:

- Reflect on their own perspectives related to digital health messages.
- Analyze how new media delivers digital health messages to the public and determine the level of evidence provided.
- Apply course content to educate a community of interest on a health concern.

Learners meet these course and section-specific objectives through three main course assignments – meme/image analysis, traditional research paper, and multimodal writing project (creation of podcast or infographic). Additional written assignments such as writer's notebook (reflective writing through journaling), journal club, proposal and progress forms, annotated bibliography, and structured peer reviews, provided scaffolding throughout the course.

Assignment 1: Meme/Image Analysis (Weeks 1–5)

In my FYW course, we prepare for this assignment right away. We discuss personal views of health, wellness, and new media in our first class meeting. To prepare for our second meeting, learners read research that explores the impact of new media on these areas. We also learn about Beaufort's knowledge domains (2007) and Ball et al.'s (2022) understanding of multimodal design. Classroom activities that day engage students through small group work that helps them summarize and critically analyze the assigned readings.

In the remaining meetings during the first two weeks of the course, learners collaboratively analyze the modes of health-related memes/images that they find online. Afterwards, learners select and analyze a meme that represents a health concern that interests them. I encourage them to consider each of the five modes in multimodal communication (Ball et al., 2022, p. 14), and they write up a "traditional" paper that follows American Psychological Association (APA) style. Before the paper's due date, I teach them a peer review process (see Appendix A), and learners demonstrate that they are ready for the peer review by submitting a draft of their writing in advance. On the day of the review, learners review the rubric that I provide on a worksheet (see Appendix B) before reading their peers' papers. We use this peer review format for all remaining writing assignments in the course, which provides an opportunity to share feedback and emotional impressions with others (Blevins et al., 2015). These interactions may widen learner perspectives and resonate in their writing, encouraging the development of a variety of health literacies. Completion of the peer review process counts as class participation. I assess the final assignment submission by using a 4-point rubric to measure each criterion assessed through the peer review process. Proficient (A), Competent (B), Beginner (C), and Novice (D/F).

Assignment 2: Research Paper (Weeks 6–11)

The second major writing assignment for the course is a research paper that addresses a health concern that learners select. This assignment spans a total of six weeks from start to submission. Additional miniature assignments (e.g., development of a working timeline for the assignment, proposal form, and an annotated bibliography) occur during those six weeks to walk learners through the writing process. The working timeline was created by learners in a small group setting based on their similar writing preferences. Learners become aware of the type of writing process they gravitate towards during the first week of class, as they answer some questions when reflecting about their previous writing experiences. Learners develop a working assignment timeline based on their writing style and preferences to keep them on task to successfully craft a research paper and avoid procrastination. This small group in-class activity enables learners to customize the working timeline to best fit their writing process preferences, whether they are "heavy drafters" or "heavy revisers."

While completing their research papers, learners gain additional skills in information literacy. The university's health science librarian holds a class session on the college library and digital resources. During the library session, they learn how to perform a proper search in academic databases using keywords, subject terms, and limiters to find current literature on their individual topic as well as discern between suitable primary and secondary sources for their research paper. The quality of paper sources is reviewed by course faculty through an annotated bibliography assignment.

This assignment can extend or stand independently from assignment 1 (meme/image analysis). Learners develop a thesis statement on a public health concern, collecting a minimum of eight kinds of research and evidence that supports their thesis. Furthermore, learners must follow APA stylist conventions to provide a professional call for action in the form of clinical practice, education, research, or policy development.

Last, I frame course meetings to monitor learners' progress on their research paper and offer constructive feedback. Learners work independently to produce a draft of particular paper sections. Learners share drafts with their peers and independently read them before providing written feedback using the peer review process outlined above (Appendix A). This process of peer review is repeated at various points throughout the paper development concentrating on the following sections: introduction, thesis/purpose statement, body of paper considerations, conclusion, abstract, and citations.

Assignment 3 (Weeks 12–15)

The last four weeks are dedicated to the final course assignment, a multimodal writing project. Specifically, learners create a public service announcement (PSA) in the form of either a visual infographic or radio podcast. A PSA is a short informational clip that raises awareness about their health concern (PennState Teaching and Learning with Technology, 2020). This style of communication is effective in communicating facts about an important issue in a manner that is likely to elicit an emotion and draw attention from the audience.

Learners create a PSA on the health concern that they wrote about in their research paper for members of the college community. If desired, learners may specify a particular audience that resides in the college community (i.e., faculty members, female athletes, business club, etc.). As learners await feedback on their submitted research papers, I have them review their individual research papers and determine which section could be transformed into a health message. Learners meet with me individually to review their PSA and discuss their ideas regarding the context of the health message as well as the digital medium that would be used to deliver the health message to the targeted audience. Learners prepare for this meeting by filling out a project proposal form (Appendix C). This document can facilitate communication during the meeting by offering a starting point and ensuring that learners have thought critically about their PSA. The project proposal form requires six responses pertaining to the topic focus, intended audience, brief description of the message, digital genre, and current or expected challenges.

Overview of the Multimodal "Writing" Process

Both infographics and podcasts are designed using the 4P process that consists of four steps – pitch, produce, publish, and promote (Groller, 2020). The proposal form mentioned previously not only assists learners as they Pitch the idea to their faculty members. It also serves as a planning guide to help them anticipate workflow and a potential timeline.

Learners then begin to Produce their multimedia products. To start, they create a storyboard that sketches out what the end product will contain. (Storyboards are a repository for multiple design elements – drawings, images, sounds, or text – which support communicating the intended message.) I encourage learners to consider the five modes of communication previously described by Ball and colleagues (2022). Once the multimodal writing project is produced, learners Publish their work on paper or online.

Learners take time to develop a dissemination plan. Planning not only prevents the project from becoming a "one hit wonder," but also enables the final step – Promote. In this final phase, the multimedia project is shared widely through intentional execution through various platforms.

Focused Class Sessions

Learners need to understand the basics about infographics and podcasts before they can effectively choose the digital genre for their PSA. Thus, during the first week of the project, we dedicate an entire class session to infographics and another session for podcast design. These class sessions guide learners through the history and purpose of the genres, orient them to the 4P process, and familiarize them with software programs that could assist with their project design, such as Apple Keynote or Microsoft PowerPoint. Either of these options provides a blank canvas for learners to design infographics without limitations. For learners who may not be so artistically inclined, I highlight third-party apps that serve as template repositories (e.g., Canva). These template programs provide some structure with respect to positioning and color schemes and give learners the opportunity to focus on textual content and other modes of communication. Apple's GarageBand was used on iPad during the podcast design class. If you do not have or like using GarageBand, you can find other third-party apps such as Anchor on your tablet or hand-held device.

Copyright Laws

When developing multimodal assignments, educators and learners need to consider copyright laws for images and sounds. Our health science librarian conducted a class session on copyright law and the Fair Use Act. If you are unfamiliar with the Fair Use Act, you may find the checklist (found on p. 124) in the third edition of Kenneth Crews's book, *Copyright law for librarians and educators,* useful. Review of these foundational principles spirited the next exercise of reviewing free and paid image and sound sources such as Creative Commons, Public Domain Music, and Audio Archive, and more. Learners need to reference these appropriately on/in their project to meet the course expectations of adhering to APA style.

Assessment and Outcomes

I grade this multimodal writing assignment based on several areas regardless of the chosen delivery method – infographic or podcast. First, I award points for how well prepared the learner was to meet and pitch their project idea. Perfection is not expected, but rather deep thought in answering the project proposal form and articulating their idea is. Second, I consider the production of their project, with respect to the learner, who used the storyboard to design an effective multimodal writing project. Third, I take into account a written narrative (2 pages maximum), in which the learner reflects on their project and explains the design choices they made. Lastly, learners present their final product in a digital showcase. As an instructor, I give feedback one more time and once the learner makes those final edits, they submit their project for possible publication in either the university newspaper (infographics) or radio station (podcasts).

In three course offerings, 50 publishable products (29 infographics and 21 podcasts) have been created over a 15-week semester. These multimodal creations cover a variety of topics from cyberbullying suicide and sleep deprivation to vaping and obesity. The university newspaper has published most infographics created in the course the semester after the course ended. The university radio station has featured podcasts in their own segment twice at the end of the semester. Both publishing outlets allow students to be a producer of health information, and they can cite this publication and/or presentation on their curricula vitae.

End-of-semester course evaluations have suggested that most learners became more confident in their writing skills as they wrote two formal papers and completed a multimedia project that is deeply rooted in health literacies. They appreciated that each assignment had meaning and built upon each other as it provided a writing portfolio of how they can write about the same topic in multiple ways. Last, the course prompted learners to examine and create new media as health experts in training. Learners started to naturally self-reflect on how they engage with new media as consumers of health information and share their experiences in the classroom.

Conclusion

This chapter shared how I, an assistant but now associate professor of nursing, designed a FYW course with assignments that expose learners to not only traditional but new media forms that are often seen in public settings. To take the assignments like these to the next level, consider working with clients outside of your institution (as Michael Klein demonstrates in Chapter 5) or applying principles of usability (as Kirk St. Amant discusses in Chapter 11).

Health communication today will require writers to take on the role of the educator at one point in time, and FYW programs can provide students with rich opportunities to develop their health literacies – informational, digital, and rhetorical. In these efforts, health-disciplined faculty can make valuable contributions. If such an opportunity is not available in your institution or you are ready to move beyond the writing studies atmosphere, I urge you to review your course curricula and consider where opportunities may lie to actively engage learners in writing and new media practices by combing multimodal projects with their discipline-specific course content.

Acknowledgment of Funding

The multimodal assignment development for this course was supported by the Andrew W. Mellon Foundation, Digital Pedagogy Humanities Course Faculty Development on April 28, 2016.

References

Askehave, I., & Nielsen, A. E. (2005). Digital genres: A challenge to traditional genre theory. *Information Technology & People*, 18(2), 120–141.

American Library Association. (1989). Presidential committee on information literacy: Final report. Chicago, Illinois: American Library Association. Available at: https://www.ala.org/acrl/publications/whitepapers/presidential

Ball, C., & Charlton, C. (2015). All writing is multimodal. In L. Adler-Kassner & E. Wardle (Eds.), *Naming what we know-threshold concepts of writing studies* (pp. 42–43), Utah State University Press.

Bailey. (2020). TikTok, It's here. *Ragtrader, May/June 2020*, 18–21. Retrieved from https://search.informit.org/doi/epdf/10.3316/informit.258774723460334

Ball, C., Sheppard, J., & Arola, K. (2022). *Writer/designer: A guide to making multimodal projects* (3rd ed.). MacMillian Learning.

Beaufort, A. (2007). *College writing and beyond-A new framework for university writing instruction.* Utah State University Press. http://compositionforum.com/issue/26/college-writing-beyond-appendix1.pdf

Beaufort, A. C. (2012). Writing and beyond: Five years later. *Composition Forum*, 26, 1–13. Retrieved on May 31, 2020 from http://compositionforum.com/issue/26/college-writing-beyond.php

Blevins, S. B., Riche, S. W., & Carpenter, R. G. (2015). Designing scholarly multimodal texts: A peer review process. *The Peer Review* (0). http://thepeerreview-iwca.org/issues/issue-0/designing-scholarly-multimodal-texts-a-peer-review-process/

Bradshaw, M. J., & Porter, S. (2017). Infographics-A new tool for the nursing classroom. *Nurse Educator*, 42(2), 57–59. doi:10.1097/NNE.0000000000000316

Bronstein, L. (2017). *Examples of Digital Genres.* Retrieved July 11 from https://laurenbronsteincom.wordpress.com/2017/02/04/examples-of-digital-genres/

Cantens, B. (2020). *Moravian College's Transition to Online Teaching.* Retrieved January 3 from https://www.moravian.edu/news/transition-to-online-teaching

Chicca, J., & Chunta, K. (2020). Engaging students with visual stories: Using infographics in nursing education. *Teaching & Learning in Nursing*, 15, 32–36. 10.1016/j.teln.2019.09.003

Cope, B., & Kalantzis, M. (2009). "Multiliteracies": New literacies, new learning. *Pedagogies: An International Journal*, 4(3), 164–195. doi 10.1080/15544800903076044

Corr, M. (2019a). *Moravian College Joins the New American Colleges and Universities-Consortium Includes Small to Midsize Colleges Nationwide.* Retrieved January 3 from https://www.moravian.edu/NAC%26U-Membership#.Xs0pIi_MzOQ

Corr, M. (2019b). *Moravian College to Provide a MacBook and iPad to Every Incoming Undergraduate Student Upon Enrollment.* Retrieved January 3 from https://www.moravian.edu/macbook-ipad-enrollment#.Xs0rJC_MzOQ

DataReportal. (2021, April-a). *Digital 2021 April Global Statshot Report.* Retrieved July 11 from https://datareportal.com/reports/digital-2021-april-global-statshot

DataReportal. (2021, April-b). *Social Media Use Around the World.* Retrieved July 11 from https://datareportal.com/social-media-users

Fodrey, C., & Hassay, C. (2021). Piloting WEC as a context-responsive writing research initiative. In C. M. Anson & Pamela Flash, Copy Edited by Don Donahue, & Designed by Mike Palmquist (Eds.), *Writing-enriched curricula: Models of faculty-driven and departmental transformation* (pp. 167–180). The WAC Clearinghouse; University Press of Colorado. 10.37514/PER-B.2021.1299.2.07

Fodrey, C., Mikovits, M., Hassay, C., & Yozell, E. (2019). Activity theory as tool for WAC program development: Organizing first-year writing and writing-enriched curriculum systems. *Composition Forum*, 42. https://compositionforum.com/issue/42/moravian.php

Groller, K. (2018). Analyzing social media imagery for health messages. *Journal of Nursing Education*, 57(3), 191–192. 10.3928/01484834-20180221-15

Groller, K. (2020). *Creating visual health messages-A focus on infographic creation.* Apple Books. https://books.apple.com/us/book/creating-visual-health-messages/id1498255428

Groller, K., Adamshick, P., & Petre, K. (2020). Embracing evidence-based nursing and informational literacy through an innovative undergraduate collaborative project. *International Journal of Nursing Education Scholarship*, 17(1). 10.1515/ijnes-2019-0138

Guslyakova, A., Guslyakova, N., Nigmatzyanova, Y., Rudneva, M., & Valeeva, N. (2018, March 5–7). New media genres and their impact on the professional development of university students in the modern digital epoch. INTED2018 Conference, pp. 9680–9685. https://www.academia.edu/38799448/NEW_MEDIA_GENRES_AND_THEIR_IMPACT_ON_THE_PROFESSIONAL_DEVELOPMENT_OF_UNIVERSITY_STUDENTS_IN_THE_MODERN_DIGITAL_EPOCH

Lynch (2017). *What is digital literacy? The Tech Edvocate.* Retrieved from https://www.thetechedvocate.org/what-is-digital-literacy/

National Institute on Aging. (2022). *Online health information: Is it reliable?* Retrieved January 3 from https://www.nia.nih.gov/health/online-health-information-it-reliable

New American Colleges and Universities (NACU). (2020). *NACU Campuses.* Retrieved January 3 from https://nacu.edu/institutions/

PennState Teaching and Learning with Technology. (2020). *Public Service Announcement.* Penn State University. Retrieved July 11 from https://mediacommons.psu.edu/2017/02/14/public-service-announcement/

Pew Research Center. (2021 April 7). *Social Media Use in 2021 Fact Sheet.* Retrieved October 25 from http://www.pewinternet.org/fact-sheet/social-media/

Prybutok, G., & Ryan, S. (2015). Social media-the key to health information access for 18- to 30-year-old college students. *Computers, Informatics, Nursing (CIN),* 33(4), 132–141. 10.1097/CIN.0000000000000147

Rattan, J. (2019). *101 Types of Digital Content. Zazzle Media.* Retrieved July 11 from https://www.zazzlemedia.co.uk/blog/digital-content-types/#gref

Schnarr, A. L. (2018). Rhetorical literacy and first year composition [Doctoral Dissertation]. University of California Riverside Doctor of Philosophy in English. Retrieved from https://escholarship.org/uc/item/8cn6g42t

World Health Organization (WHO). (2020). *State of the World's Nursing.* World Health Organization. https://www.who.int/publications-detail/nursing-report-2020

Additional Reading

Burke, J. (2018). Infographics for info pros. *Online Searcher,* 42(1), 51–56. https://www.infotoday.com/OnlineSearcher/Articles/Features/Infographics-for-Info-Pros-123086.shtml

Chicca, J., & Chunta, K. (2020). Engaging students with visual stories: Using infographics in nursing education. *Teaching & Learning in Nursing,* 15, 32–36. doi: 10.1016/jteln.2019.09.003

Dunlap, J. C., & Lowenthal, P. R. (2016). Getting graphic about infographics: Design lessons learned from popular infographics. *Journal of Visual Literacy,* 35(1), 42–59. doi: 10.1080/1051144X.2016.1205832

Groller, K. (2020). *Creating visual health messages-A focus on infographic creation.* Apple Books. Retrieved on May 31, 2020 from https://books.apple.com/us/book/creating-visual-health-messages/id1498255428

Royal, K. D., & Erdmann, K. M. (2017). Evaluating the readability levels of medical infographic materials for public consumption. *Journal of Visual Communication in Medicine,* 41(3), 99–102. doi: 10.80/17453054.2018.1476059

Appendix A: Teaching the Peer Review Process

1. Learners share draft of assignment in Dropbox prior to class meeting.
2. Instructor develops and shares peer review worksheet. Assignment specific criteria is added to the general peer review worksheet under the criteria "genre style & formatting."
3. Learners begin the peer review process by reading assignment drafts. First read occurs without learners making any comments or corrections. Second read permits comments and corrections (on assignment), and reflections (peer review form).
4. Peer reviewer navigates draft and peer review worksheet to assess criteria and provide constructive feedback.
5. Learners share feedback. First, in written form and then through verbal exchange.

Appendix B: Peer Review Criteria

Each category is ranked using the following marks: Meets expectations (5), Needs Improvement (3) or Below Expectations (0)

1. Introduction: How does the first paragraph introduce both the paper's topic and the writer's approach? Is the first sentence attention-getting and relevant to the topic?
2. Thesis Statement: Sentence that shares the main idea or premise to the piece of writing.
3. Body Paragraphs: Does each body paragraph contains a topic sentence (or implied main idea), sentences within each paragraph build and connect to the main idea? Does the last sentence summarize (conclude) the discussion of the paragraph?
4. Structure & Organization: Is the overall paper organized in a way that is easy to follow? Is each paragraph logically sequenced with transitions used to link ideas together when appropriate? Does anything appear to be out of place or artificially connected? If so, share your findings.
5. Conclusion: Is the conclusion of the paper summarized in one paragraph the essence of the paper in a memorable way? Did the author restate the main point (thesis/purpose) without being said verbatim? Remember, no sources or new information should be presented.
6. Genre/Style & Formatting: Assignment-specific criteria are provided. For example, when considering the meme/image analysis assignment criteria could be: Has the author conducted a thorough analysis of design elements of a visual health message available on new media? Was APA formatting (7th edition) used with adherence to Title page, reference page and citation style formatting guides? Was proper in-text and reference format used.

7. Grammar/Sentence Structure Concerns: Is the paper is free from grammar, punctuation, spelling or word usage problems? Did the author write adequately (think if paragraph formation, sentence structure, correct comma/semicolon use, spellcheck, was executed with quality)?
8. Resource Creditability: How is the information provided supported? Do references or sources come from a creditable source that has gone through a peer-reviewed process? If not, rationale is provided and justified for why the source is used in academic writing.

Appendix C: Project Proposal Form

Name of Designer/Author:

	Ask Yourself …	Write Down Your Project Thoughts Here …
Topic Focus	*What is your selected health concern?*	
Intended Audience	*Who is your main audience? Why did you choose them?*	
Intended Message	*What message do you hope to communicate to the selected audience? Why this message?*	
Brief Description	*Include an outline of areas you plan to address digitally. Share storyboard draft or sketchnote if available.*	
Digital Genre	*What modality (infographic, podcast, song, video) will you use for the development of your idea?*	
Current or expected challenges experienced	*Are you planning on or having difficulties? If so, what are they and how are you planning to trouble shooting them?*	

2

TEACHING CRITICAL THINKING FOR CRITICAL HEALTH LITERACIES: A PROBLEM-BASED WRITING APPROACH

Kasey Larson, Jill Paterson-Charles, and Karina Daniel

Health literacy includes "the evolving skills and competencies needed to … make educated choices, reduce health risks, and improve quality of life" (Zarcadoolas et al., 2003, p. 119). This elaboration points to the importance of critical thinking. In this chapter, we argue that critical health literacies, as an extension of critical thinking, is vital for undergraduates, whether they enter the health professions, become health communicators, or otherwise engage extensively with health-related information.

This chapter outlines the importance of critical thinking skills and their connections to critical health literacies. To make our abstract discussion more concrete, we illustrate a problem-based writing approach that focuses on a Proposal Paper. Through the different stages of the writing process, students at our institution identify a One Health problem and propose a practical, reasoned solution to help solve it. The assignment helps students develop multiple critical health literacy competencies including:

- Analyzing, evaluating, and synthesizing ideas;
- Identifying and articulating the significance of problems; and
- Proposing practical solutions to current One-Health problems.

In Appendix 1, we share evidence of critical thinking and health literacy competencies within a sample student paper that we have annotated.

Critical Health Literacies

Traditionally, health literacy has referred to individuals acting for their own benefit, which is of course important. But critical health literacies go further:

DOI: 10.4324/9781003316770-4

critical health literacies account for finding, understanding, and using health information to benefit others – much like Freire's concept of community development where citizens recognize health issues, critically dialogue about them, and engage in the decision-making process. This inclusive process allows individuals to develop "an understanding of the determinants and the policy context of health, an understanding of opportunities to challenge these determinants and policy and motivation and actual action at a political and social level" (Sykes et al., 2013, p. 5). Based on these concepts, Sykes et al. (2013) suggested that critical health literacies can be developed through education as students critically appraise information that has relevance to health (p. 2).

Some of the higher-order thinking skills required for critical health literacies align with the American Psychological Association's definition of critical thinking: "purposeful, self-regulatory judgment which results in interpretation, analysis, evaluation, and inference, as well as explanation of the evidential, conceptual, methodological, criteriological, or contextual considerations upon which that judgment is based" (Facione, 1990, p.2). Each of the six critical thinking cognitive skills can be divided into subskills, which we describe in Table 2.1.

We believe that these critical thinking skills can support the development of critical health literacies, including in undergraduate writing classrooms.

Teaching Critical Thinking for Critical Health Literacies through Undergraduate Writing Instruction

Teaching critical thinking for critical health literacies requires methods of content delivery that encourage students to process the material on a deep level (Oyler & Romanelli, 2014). One way to do so, including in health-related contexts (see, e.g., Oja, 2011), is through problem-based learning (PBL). Duch and colleagues (2001) explain that in PBL, "complex, real-world problems are used to motivate students to identify and research the concepts and principles they need to know to work through those problems" (p. 6). Facing real-world problems, students take on the role of "professional problem solvers" (Stepien et al., 1993, p. 338), who must make use of conceptual reasoning and understanding, systems and organizers, scientific observation and research, resource identification and evaluation, collaboration, and ongoing authentic assessments (Burruss, 1999). PBL additionally encourages student reflection, curiosity, and exploration, along with truth seeking and analyticity (Tiwari et al., 2006). In all this, teachers take on the role of "guides on the side" rather than "sages on the stage."

A related, student-centered way to develop critical thinking skills for critical health literacies is through meaningful writing assignments. Students' performance on writing assignments can make visible their abilities to reason (Terryberry, 2005), and in turn, the process of writing can improve the students' reasoning. Studies have investigated the link between writing and

TABLE 2.1 Critical thinking cognitive skills and sub-skills (Facione, 1990, p. 6)

Cognitive Skills	Sub-skills	Descriptions
Interpretation	Categorizing	Grouping information meaningfully
	Decoding significance	Identifying, understanding, and describing meaning
	Clarifying meaning	Paraphrasing and making understanding clear.
Analysis	Examining ideas	Explaining terms, comparing information, and determining and breaking down issues
	Identifying arguments	Identifying reasons in support of claims or opinions.
	Analyzing arguments	Dissecting arguments into their various components for a complete understanding of the argument.
Evaluation	Assessing claims	Determining the credibility of information
	Assessing arguments	Evaluating the reasoning behind an argument
Inference	Querying evidence	Determining propositions that need support and then developing a plan to find that support
	Conjecturing alternatives	Coming up with different ways of doing things like solving problems or reaching goals.
	Drawing conclusions	Using reason and evidence to determine the most appropriate conclusions.
Explanation	Stating results	Effectively articulating one's reasoning
	Justifying procedures	Providing rationales for claims, analyses, inferences, or interpretations.
	Presenting arguments	Providing reasons in support of a claim
Self-regulation	Self-examination	Reflecting on one's reasoning and beliefs and what has contributed to these beliefs
	Self-correction	Correcting the errors identified during self-regulation.

critical thinking in science classes and overall, these studies have shown that incorporating writing of some kind improved students' critical thinking competencies (Daempfle, 2002; Quitadamo & Kurtz, 2007; Stephenson & Sadler-McKnight, 2016). Writing assignments can have more general effects on learning as well. According to the National Commission on Writing's (2003) report, writing does not just demonstrate students' knowledge, but it is a valuable tool to help them comprehend what they know (see also Klein & Boscolo, 2016). Part of the reason is the metacognition involved in many writing tasks, which encourages students to not only recognize and order their thoughts, but also reflect on, analyze, and evaluate their own ideas. Harnessing these advantages, problem-based writing, as a sub-field of PBL, gives students opportunities to develop critical thinking qualities as they solve problems and also write about problem solving.

Not all our undergraduate students will enter the health professions of course. But for those who do, problem-based writing may be particularly useful. Problem-based writing, which often involves research, may help students attain the communication competencies demanded by their profession, such as conveying succinct ideas, translating scientific data, and applying information to policy changes that can impact patient outcomes (Malik, 2017; Medical Schools Council, 2008; Sharma 2010). Terryberry (2005) further suggests that instructors teach writing for personal ethical reasons and presents writing as crucial preparation for the healthcare industry. Indeed, studies have shown that critical thinking skills, which problem-based writing can promote, can support students' performance on certification examinations (Ross et al., 2013) and clinical decision-making (Heidari & Ebrahimi, 2016), among other areas. However, like much of the general public, aspiring health professionals, too, may have inadequate levels of health literacy, critical and otherwise (e.g., Moretti et al., 2021). At St. George's University (SGU), we recognized these challenges and designed a communication course that uses problem-based writing and health-related information to give students a strong foundation in the critical thinking health competencies that they will undoubtably need as professionals.

Academic Context

Communication for the Health Professions II (CHP II) is a mandatory intensive communications writing course delivered in the final term of the undergraduate preprofessional programs (premedical and pre-veterinary) at SGU. SGU was founded in 1976 on the Caribbean island of Grenada. SGU started as a medical school and has since expanded to offer degrees in public health, veterinary medicine, arts and sciences, and business. The School of Medicine is the core of the institution. The institution's students and faculty originate from over 150 countries, and between 1981 and 2022 SGU has contributed over 19,000 physicians to the global physician workforce. SGU's preclinical and pre-veterinary program is currently housed in the School of Arts and Sciences, and CHP II is considered one of the fundamental courses undergraduate students must complete to begin their journey toward medical school.

CHP II teaches academic argumentative writing and critical thinking skills, taking a problem-based writing approach. Before completing CHP II, students must successfully pass Communication for the Health Professions I, where they develop foundational academic and research writing skills. The average class size is approximately 60 and the student population is significantly diverse, with students from North America, Asia, Africa, the Caribbean, and Europe. The course is team-taught by a group of 3–4 instructors with each instructor working closely with a cohort of 15–20 students. Instructors support their cohort of students throughout the semester, providing intensive feedback and guidance.

They work closely with students to develop their proposals writing over 6–8 weeks, meeting with them twice a week for 75 minutes per class.

The course is student-centered, collaborative, and integrative, applying principles of PBL. Additionally, to encourage student participation and interest, the course promotes "One Health," which is defined as "a collaborative, multisectoral, and transdisciplinary approach—working at the local, regional, national, and global levels—with the goal of achieving optimal health outcomes recognizing the interconnection between people, animals, plants, and their shared environment" (Center for Disease Control and Prevention, 2022). One Health describes human health as closely linked to the health of animals and the environment, and advocates for a comprehensive approach: addressing animal and human health as well as environmental problems. Issues such as vector-borne diseases, environmental contamination, zoonotic diseases, and diseases in food animals fall within the One Health domain. Although the concept of the interconnected nature of health is not new (see, e.g., the Lalonde report mentioned in the introductory chapter), recent developments such as climate change, the expansion of humans into new geographic areas, and the greater movement of animals, humans, and products over international boundaries have made this concept more relevant. COVID-19 was quickly spread because of this ease of movement. Furthermore, it was caused by the zoonotic virus, SARS-CoV-2.

In CHP II, our class materials and activities draw from recent relevant One Health domains and, through its interdisciplinary scientific focus, interests both pre-medical and pre-veterinary students. Specifically, we enact One Health through a Proposal Paper.

Problem-based Writing Assignment

The Proposal Paper is an argumentative essay in which students propose a solution (or partial solution) to a One Health issue. Past Proposal Paper topics have focused on tackling the invasive lionfish population in Grenada; reducing malaria cases in Lagos, Nigeria; and addressing the outbreak of the water-borne disease Leptospirosis in Puerto Rico. In this paper, students are required to evaluate the significant issues surrounding their topic, offer a practical, original solution, justify their stance, and outline the key steps moving forward. The paper also takes students through the various stages of writing process, applying critical thinking skills, while immersing themselves in topics that are relevant and authentic to their overall learning experience.

As Rank and Pool (2014) stated, "though most instructors care deeply about student writing, they often give little attention to the part of the writing process over which they maintain complete control: the assignment itself" (p.675). Thus, to help students accomplish the complex tasks entailed in the assignment, we provide detailed guidelines to assist them in the various stages of the writing process. The importance of assignment guidelines is often overlooked, and the result can be muddled, ambiguous instructions that mislead students or confuse them about the overall goals of the task. The guidelines are crucial for not only introducing and explaining the assignment but also for providing continual guidance for students at various stages in the assignment when they may need a refresher. Like Çavdar and Doe (2012), we believe that "through well-designed writing assignments, instructors can encourage students to reconsider concepts, critically evaluate assumptions, and undertake substantive revisions" (p. 298).

The guidelines provide a clear description of expectations. They begin with the general goal of the assignment, due dates for smaller tasks associated with the assignment, word count, percentage of course grade, and required sources. Next, the objectives for the assignment are clarified using precise verbs that identify discrete tasks. Students are expected to evaluate a One Health problem, identify a practical solution (their proposal) to the problem, provide valid reasons for it, and develop at least three steps involved in accomplishing their plan. Potential misconceptions of the assignment are also noted in that section. For example, students are reminded that they are required to create one solution, not multiple solutions for their issue. After this, some finer details of the assignment are included, such as an acronym to help students decide on a topic for their paper, the major stages of the paper, and a suggested process for writing the paper. Attached at the end of the assignment guidelines is the rubric which is also useful for clarifying the expectations of the paper, maintaining a standard and consistency with the papers (see Çavdar & Doe, 2012), and allowing students to assess their progress as writers.

Proposal Paper Components

Because the Proposal Paper is a complex assignment that engages various levels of problem-based writing, the assignment is broken in multiple parts, as Baglione (2008) suggests. The major components of the Proposal Paper are covered explicitly in the course through in-class activities and homework assignments. The activities help to introduce and explain key concepts in the paper and provide practice with those tasks. The breakdown below demonstrates the major components of the Proposal Paper and various opportunities for students to develop their "critical thinking for critical health literacies."

Evaluate a One Health One Medicine problem

This section of the paper requires students to (1) survey the literature on their focus problem, (2) determine the significant issues around the topic in a global context but ultimately narrowed to their localized issue, and (3) argue the significance and extent of the problem by evaluating the One Health connections, consequences, and implications. These tasks encourage students to employ many of the 16 critical thinking sub-skills identified by the APA (Facione, 1990) to fully capture the significance of a One Health One Medicine issue and its associated arguments – developing competencies needed for critical health literacies. For example, for students to be successful they need to first categorize their problems to ensure they fit into a One Health framework. They need to examine ideas, clarify meaning, and decode significance through a detailed description of their One Health problem. They then need to query evidence to support their justification of the problem (justifying procedures). Students are required to use credible evidence in the evaluation of their problem, which showcases their capacity to assess claims. They must also understand the links between ideas to be able to make meaningful, reasonable connections across disciplines.

Identify a Practical Solution (or Partial Solution) to the Problem

This component is the foundation for students' papers. The solution they propose should be feasible, original, and relevant. To arrive at a suitable solution, students must assess the ineffectiveness of current measures addressing the issue, review effective strategies for similar issues outside of their focus location, create an original proposal that feasibly applies to their context, and determine which entity/organization(s) should implement the proposal. For this section, students are required to analyze and synthesize evidence and use reasoning skills to fill gaps in the literature. These steps allow students to practice critical thinking. Specifically, students are first focusing on conjecturing alternatives to identify various solutions to their One Health problem and then they are drawing conclusions to determine the "best" solution for their problem based on evidence and real-world limitations. Students are also providing justification for their steps (justifying procedures) and reasoning in support of these steps in their solution (presenting arguments). This aspect of the paper aligns with Sykes et al.'s (2013) notion of critical health literacy and the importance of using health information for decision-making and action.

Justify the Proposal with Valid Reasons

This component is closely linked to the proposed solution as students evaluate the effectiveness of their solution and develop sound reasons why it is an ideal proposal for that issue. Also associated with the justification is the counter-argument section where students are encouraged to entertain potential opposing views to their proposal, validate them, but reaffirm their stance. By evaluating their proposal and conflicting arguments, students are encouraged to use critical thinking skills to reflect on the validity of their own ideas and assumptions and create, appraise, and defend arguments showcasing their capacity in the critical thinking subskills of presenting arguments, justifying procedures, conjecturing alternatives, and drawing conclusions. The justification also requires students to demonstrate "an understanding of the determinants and the policy context of health, an understanding of opportunities to challenge these determinants and policy and motivation and actual action at apolitical and social level" (Sykes et al., 2013, p. 5), an essential part of critical health literacies.

Develop at Least 3 Details or Steps Involved In Accomplishing the Proposal

Developing practical, feasible steps and supporting them with evidence and analysis requires students to make connections to real-life experiences, limitations, and the reality of implementing a proposal. In this section, students must employ analytical and critical thinking skills to break big ideas into concrete tasks that map out their proposals in a practical way. In their detailed description of their steps, students must employ the critical thinking sub-skills of stating results, justifying procedures, and presenting arguments so that the reader can clearly understand how to implement the solution.

The Writing Process

In addition to breaking down the components of the Proposal Paper, we guide students through the writing process. As a result, the paper is completed in multiple stages with ongoing feedback and assessments at each point. The major parts of the writing process engaged in this course are discovery/investigation, prewriting, drafting, revising, and final submission. It must be noted that the writing process is often more cyclical than linear, meaning that students may need to repeat certain stages as they move forward. This section will elaborate on both why and how we take students through the writing process.

Feedback

First, we wish to emphasize the importance of feedback. Feedback is an essential part of the writing process, and if effectively integrated at each stage, it can significantly impact the quality of the final product. In fact, ongoing oral and written feedback on students' assignments is crucial in sharpening their critical thinking skills (e.g., self-examination and self-correction) and overall writing abilities (Çavdar & Doe, 2012). As Mehta and Al-Mahrooqi (2015) stated, "continuous practice, both oral and written, provides opportunities for students to develop their critical thinking abilities as they become more successful in incorporating nuanced and critical ideas into their academic writings" (p. 1). Thus, in our course, instructors and peers provide a combination of oral and written feedback at each stage in the writing process, encouraging students to refine their verbal and written communication.

Because feedback is a central part of the course, it is strategically addressed in course content and used as the primary tool to facilitate students' progress throughout the term. As a foundational principle, the course strives to expose students to the importance of feedback and develop an appreciation for it in their professional careers. As a result, class time is devoted to describing feedback, highlighting its benefits, and demonstrating effective and ineffective feedback. This is done within the framework of the growth mindset to relieve some of the tension and apprehension students experience regarding feedback. We also describe our major feedback principles to students and underscore that it is one tool to help improve their writing, among other tools used in the course. They learn how to provide effective peer feedback and read and incorporate our feedback as they see fit. Specifically, with regard to written feedback, we use guided peer feedback. This is an active learning tool that allows students to assume the instructors' role and employ their critical thinking abilities to assess their peers' papers, which in turn refines the reviewer's thinking processes. Instructors, however, provide more comprehensive feedback that challenges students to think critically about their revisions. The feedback places an emphasis on deep-level feedback that guides students towards making revisions without instructing them on what revisions to make.

As a teaching team, we aim to provide targeted, consistent, sensitive, prompt, specific, and instructive feedback that inspires students to continue honing skills, but also challenges them to make revisions that improve the impact of their work. Because students enter our class with a range of academic experiences, diverse cultural backgrounds, and various levels of familiarity with North American English, we use feedback as our main avenue for addressing individual issues with critical thinking and scientific writing. (For more on linguistic and cultural considerations, see Chapter 9, where Catherine E. Morelli discusses her work with cultural health navigators.) Students receive personalized and targeted feedback to help them progress at a suitable pace for their levels, and in instances where they require additional assistance not offered in the course, we refer them to supplementary writing support programs in our department and encourage them to regularly meet with their cohort leader.

In general, our feedback prioritizes the major issues in the paper as a focal point and largely revolves around big picture ideas, critical analysis, and logical sequencing, in accordance with the assignment guidelines. Although we may point to patterns of grammatical issues in students' papers, they are mostly required to address mechanical and editing issues through Grammarly and other course resources provided. Since students often place an inordinate emphasis on grades, we make feedback the primary element of focus: each stage of the process is graded on effort and students use feedback and highlights we provide on the rubric to assess how they can improve. Only the final submission is graded on performance. Our cohort leaders are also readily available to students who wish to book appointments and receive additional feedback where necessary.

In the following sections, we illustrate how, applying these feedback practices, we guide students through the different components of the paper. (For another perspective on peer review, see Chapter 1.)

Discovery and Investigation (1 week)

Before students engage in targeted writing activities related to their Proposal Papers, they must first acquire sufficient background knowledge on One Health and demonstrate a thorough understanding of the paper requirements. The goal of this stage is to help students activate prior knowledge, gather rudimentary data on important concepts, determine what a suitable topic looks like, and begin entertaining potential topics. Therefore, we integrate relevant instructional content and activities to prepare students for the more writing-focused stages.

Independent Activities: students read assigned One Health research articles and are instructed to note clarifying questions and begin thinking of topics within the field that make a clear interdisciplinary connection between animal, human, and/ or environmental health.

Guest Lecture: a resident One Health professional introduces One Health to the class by discussing the importance and key components of the framework; presenting real-world, relevant case studies; and providing opportunities for students to pose questions and enquire about potential topics.

Classroom Instruction: the One Health framework and its practical applications are further explored in subsequent classes. Major elements include a review of One Health concepts, how it applies in local environments, and a thorough explanation of the components and expectations. Students are also guided on selecting appropriate topics that interest them and given the opportunity to evaluate sample topics from former students. We also outline essential questions to generate ideas and capture the criteria for topic selection with the acronym "DOORS" (debatable, One Health, original, researchable, and specific).

These classes include some presentations of content but mostly focus on group activities that foster effective application of the material. For example, in one in-class activity, students are split into groups of 4–5 and given a specific One Health case study to read, evaluate, and briefly present to the class. In their presentations, they are required to answer key questions that relate to the effective development of their own topics: (1) summarize the case study and problem, (2) explain the One Health link (which disciplines are connected and how?), (3) highlight multiple issues around this topic, (4) consider a preliminary solution, or partial solution, to the problem. As students present their ideas in class, the instructors raise questions to ensure understanding and further elaborate on challenging concepts, such as selecting a narrow feasible solution.

Prewriting (2 weeks)

The prewriting phase marks the start of the writing activities. In this stage, students are encouraged to generate, develop, test, and note their ideas in various forms. It is an imperfect, messy stage where students play around with ideas and potential plans, not too concerned about creating a final, concrete product. Yet, prewriting strategies are key to improving the quality of students' writing if they are taught and meaningfully incorporated into the course (Servati, 2012). At this stage, students are deciding one major topic, narrowing their focus, and reviewing additional literature to gather data for their arguments. Prewriting can be seen as an essential part of problem-based learning where students grapple with the "messiness of the real world" (see Burruss, 1999, p. 47) while engaging what Healthy People 2030 term as the "find and understand information" component of critical health literacies (Office of Disease Prevention and Health Promotion, 2021). In this course, prewriting is done through explicit practice with brainstorming techniques in class and as part of submitted assignments.

Brain dumping: a fundamental brainstorming technique where ideas are quickly jotted down on a piece of paper or smart device and used as a basis for further development. This is a foundational tool to help students itemize what they currently know about their topics and issues they may need to address. It is also an effective classroom activity when conducted with the entire group. For example, in an online setting, asking students to brain dump what they have learned about One Health in the chat provides critical instruction and reminders from their peers.

Freewriting: writing about a specific prompt without an assigned structure, sometimes within a given time frame. One of the key tenets of freewriting is to never stop writing. Students are encouraged to keep writing even if they feel like they have nothing to say, or if their thoughts wander. The goal is to process ideas and challenge the need to write perfectly in the beginning stages of writing. This skill particularly helps students who are prone to "writer's block" and have difficulty producing work in timed settings. In CHP 2, freewriting is introduced early in the course with more casual, reflective topics, and geared more toward Proposal Paper topics later in the semester.

Concept mapping: visual representations of data in a variety of forms, including charts, graphic organizers, tables, customized designs. These can be created manually through physical sketches or digitally through freely available concept mapping software. Concept mapping, in fact, has been found to be linked to an increase in critical thinking (Atay & Karabacak, 2012; Daley et al., 1999; Wilgis & McConnell, 2008). Students who have a preference for visual processing tend to lean more toward this method. In the context of this course, students use concept maps to brainstorm in the major components of the paper in relation to their potential topics and identify crucial connections. This visual format helps to provide additional perspective on their rough ideas and tap into their creativity. When students submit their concept maps, instructors review them in a cursory manner to ensure they have a viable topic and that they demonstrate a general understanding of the topic. To make efficient use of time, we only provide essential feedback where necessary.

Preliminary vision: this tool has been customized by the CHP 2 teaching team to help students identify important aspects of the Proposal Paper and develop a rough draft of ideas. Students post their preliminary visions on a Forum platform for peer and instructor review. In this vision, they answer specific questions that encourage them to thoroughly evaluate the significance of the problem and the feasibility of their potential solution. Students are required to use the essential questions in the preliminary vision to assess their peers' posts and provide feedback on the strengths of the preliminary vision and areas for improvement. Instructors then provide a second layer of feedback, whether that's "green-lighting" the peer's feedback, correcting misguided information, or providing more details on areas of strengths and weaknesses. Because this is a short activity, it allows instructors to intervene early in the writing process and guide students accordingly. The public format of this activity allows students to learn from a variety of topics and reviews and assess their own feedbacking skills.

Outlining: a general plan of the various components in the order in which they will appear in the final product. Outlines help students delineate their ideas in each paragraph, including potential pieces of evidence, and establish a logical sequence of ideas. In CHP 2, students practice outlining as their first major submission for the Proposal Paper. At this point, they have conducted significant research on their topics and received feedback on their preliminary visions, so they are more prepared to develop an outline. Students are given the option to create their own outline (as long as it follows a logical argumentative essay format and addresses the major parts of the paper) or use the outline template instructors provide. Whichever option they choose, they are at liberty to redesign aspects of the outline to suit their preferences. They also receive detailed instructions on outlining their paper through instructional videos, activities, and official guidelines. After students submit their outlines, they engage in peer conferences to further refine their ideas and engage in the next stage of feedbacking (*see peer conferences below*).

Peer Conferences: in groups of two, students meet with their cohort leaders for 30 minutes to review their peer's outline and incorporate oral feedback from their partner and their instructor. Students are provided with a document detailing the conference guidelines and rubric to establish expectations before the meeting. They are instructed to evaluate their peer's outline based on the expectations of the paper and specific guiding questions. They are also required to highlight and justify strong elements and offer suggestions for areas of improvement. Students are required to take detailed notes as the information provided serves as their feedback for the first draft. Instructors are present to provide additional feedback and correct misconceptions and unhelpful advice. This element was introduced into the course to remedy the limitations of written feedback and ensure students were on the right track before investing their time in a fully developed argumentative essay. Peer conferences are also an effective way to conduct peer review as students not only practice critical thinking by reviewing their peer's paper but their feedback is also vetted and clarified by the instructor. In addition, students who may not receive thorough feedback from their peers still benefit as the instructor is prepared to provide relevant feedback.

Drafting (3 weeks)

Students' prewriting activities culminate into one major draft of the Proposal Paper (draft 1). At this point in the writing process, students are expected to synthesize and analyze sources to produce a coherent, reasonable argument. They have received feedback on their general plans and are expected to further craft those ideas into a well-developed argumentative essay.

In tandem with this process, course instruction focuses on reviewing essay structure and development and helps students practice expressing their ideas in paragraph form. This includes content and practice on identifying the main ideas for each paragraph; effectively incorporating evidence; developing counterarguments; and analyzing and synthesizing sources for the various parts of the essay. In the assignment guidelines, students are required to stay within a maximum word limit but not penalized for exceeding it, as the first draft is still a rough start at the final product. Instructor feedback will focus on helping the students address major issues in the essay, including underdevelopment and irrelevant information. This is the most feedback-intensive phase of the paper, as instructors provide comprehensive details on strong elements in the essay; pertinent paragraph-level comments about ways to improve individual sections; precise questions that encourage students to think critically about their information; major grammatical or mechanical issues and trends; and suggested resources for review to assist in revisions.

Despite this phase being the most feedback-intensive, we avoid overwhelming the students with too many comments and instead prioritize the most critical issues that will have maximum impact if addressed. Although the paper is graded on effort, instructors include a copy of the rubric and highlight the section in which the paper falls. Students who require significant assistance are instructed to book an appointment with their cohort leader.

Revising and Final Submission (2 weeks)

This is the culminating product that students submit to be graded based on performance and the overall expectations in the rubric. The final submission is supported in class with a series of targeted writing workshops. As instructors review draft 1, they take note of strong and weak areas in students' writing, along with short samples of effective work to demonstrate anonymously to the class. Based on the analysis of students' performance, workshops are developed to review critical concepts, show model work, and practice key skills that can improve the final products. Some of the in-class activities include group peer reviews on assigned paragraphs, application of checklists questions to assess elements of their essays, quizzes on critical misunderstandings, and evaluation of ineffective samples.

At this point in the course, we introduce full sample papers from former students. We avoid introducing sample papers before the first draft as students tend to limit their ideas and creativity to what is demonstrated in the sample papers. However, introducing them after the first draft is created allows students to solely use them as models and guides for refining their own ideas. Feedback on the final drafts is minimal as students rarely review them and are most concerned with the placement on the rubric and the grade received at that point in the term. The final comments focus on general performance, praise, and progress, and may include one or two instructional suggestions for future writing. A complete final draft Proposal Paper from a previous CHP 2 student is included in the chapter's appendices. Our annotations on this Proposal Paper highlight 13 of the 16 critical thinking sub-skills this student's sample exhibits.

Conclusion

This chapter explored the use of a problem-based writing assignment (the Proposal Paper) to develop critical thinking for critical health literacies in an undergraduate context. PBL and writing activities are methods that have shown a significant impact in developing students' disposition for and application of critical thinking skills. In the writing assignment discussed, students proposed a solution (or partial solution) to a One Health problem and completed multiple analytic, evaluative, and reflective tasks to create and refine an original, logical, and academic argument. To arrive at a final product, students worked through the various stages of the writing process and engaged in a series of instructor and peer feedback loops, both oral and written. The entire process, from the assignment guidelines to the conceptualization of a One Health problem and the integration of current research to create an effective argumentative essay, encourages students to develop and apply critical thinking skills. Applying critical thinking skills to a health problem encourages students to develop competencies for critical health literacies. Competencies such as sharing ideas succinctly;

finding, interpreting, and translating scientific data; and evaluating and using the information to impact patient outcomes are only a few of the ways that health professionals use critical health literacies to benefit the lives of others.

The implementation of this writing project for over six semesters has revealed some key ideas. First, critical thinking instruction often feels unfamiliar and unnecessary to the student population, and they find it challenging to engage in learning on a deeper level while making meaningful connections across domains. However, it is also noted that the Proposal Paper develops students' disposition to think critically over time with continued practice and activities geared to elicit their cognitive capacities. Additionally, writing (particularly through the writing process with timely and relevant feedback) is an effective way to help students process their thoughts and develop more logical and comprehensive thinking patterns. These skills not only improve writing capabilities but develop students' critical health literacies, which is highly likely to positively impact medical practice and patient care. Because health professionals create and use health information regularly, critical health literacies, as an extension of critical thinking, are essential. Writing the Proposal Paper moves SGU's aspiring health professionals significantly closer towards making educated choices, reducing health risks, and improving the quality of life for themselves and for those in their care. Capacity in these aspects of critical health literacies is vital for all undergraduates and not strictly aspiring health professionals.

This evaluation of a problem-based writing assignment shows the significance of integrating explicit critical thinking training and writing in undergraduate medical preprofessional programs, and calls for further research, specifically an assessment of students' critical thinking skills prior to and post-completion of the Proposal Paper.

References

Atay, S., & Karabacak, Ü. (2012). Care plans using concept maps and their effects on the critical thinking dispositions of nursing students. *International Journal of Nursing Practice*, 18(3), 233–239. 10.1111/j.1440-172x.2012.02034.x

Baglione, L. (2008). Doing good and doing well: Teaching research-paper writing by unpacking the paper. *PS: Political Science & Politics*, 41(3), 595–602. http://www.jstor.org/stable/20452254

Burruss, J. D. (1999). Problem-based learning. *Science Scope*, 22(6), 46.

Çavdar, G., & Doe, S. (2012). Learning through writing: Teaching critical thinking skills in writing assignments. *PS: Political Science & Politics*, 45(2), 298–306. 10.1017/S1049096511002137

Centers for Disease Control and Prevention. (2022). *One Health*. https://www.cdc.gov/onehealth/index.html

Daempfle, P. A. (2002). Instructional approaches for the improvement of reasoning in introductory college biology courses: A review of the research. https://files.eric.ed.gov/fulltext/ED468720.pdf

Daley, B. J., Shaw, C. A., Balistrieri, T., Glasenapp, K., & Piacentine, L. (1999). Concept maps: A strategy to teach and evaluate critical thinking. *Journal of Nursing Education*, 38(1), 42–47. https://pubmed.ncbi.nlm.nih.gov/9921788/

Duch, B. J., Groh, S. E., & Allen, D. E. (2001). *The power of problem-based learning: a practical "how to" for teaching undergraduate courses in any discipline.* Stylus Publishing, LLC.

Facione, P. A. (1990). Critical thinking: A statement of expert consensus for purposes of educational assessment and instruction (The Delphi Report). https://www.qcc.cuny.edu/socialsciences/ppecorino/CT-Expert-Report.pdf

Heidari, M., & Ebrahimi, P. (2016). Examining the relationship between critical-thinking skills and decision-making ability of emergency medicine students. *Indian Journal of Critical Care Medicine: Peer-reviewed, Official Publication of Indian Society of Critical Care Medicine*, 20(10), 581. 10.4103%2F0972-5229.192045

Klein, P. D., & Boscolo, P. (2016). Trends in research on writing as a learning activity. *Journal of Writing Research*, 7(3), 311–350. 10.17239/jowr-2016.07.03.01

Malik, B. (2017). The value of writing skills as an addition to the medical school curriculum. *Advances in Medical Education and Practice*, 8, 525. 10.2147%2FAMEP.S140585

Medical Schools Council. (2008). *Statement on the Core Values and Attributes Needed to Study Medicine: 2018 Update.* https://www.medschools.ac.uk/media/2542/statement-on-core-values-to-study-medicine.pdf

Mehta, S. R., & Al-Mahrooqi, R. (2015). Can thinking be taught? Linking critical thinking and writing in an EFL context. *RELC journal*, 46(1), 23–36. 10.1177/0033688214555356

Moretti, V., Valdi, G., Brunelli, L., Arnoldo, L., Conte, A., Masoni, M., Guelfi, M. R., & Anelli, F. (2021). e-Health Literacy among medical students. *European Journal of Public Health*, 31(Supplement_3), ckab165-145. 10.1093/eurpub/ckab165.145

Office of Disease Prevention and Health Promotion. 2021. *Health Literacy in Health People 2030.* https://health.gov/our-work/national-health-initiatives/healthy-people/healthy-people-2030/health-literacy-healthy-people-2030

Oja, K. J. (2011). Using problem-based learning in the clinical setting to improve nursing students' critical thinking: An evidence review. *Journal of Nursing Education*, 50(3), 145–151. 10.3928/01484834-20101230-10

Oyler, D. R., & Romanelli, F. (2014). The Fact of Ignorance: Revisiting the Socratic Method as a Tool for Teaching Critical Thinking. *American Journal of Pharmaceutical Education*, 78(7). 10.5688/ajpe787144

Quitadamo, I. J., & Kurtz, M. J. (2007). Learning to improve: Using writing to increase critical thinking performance in general education biology. *CBE—Life Sciences Education*, 6(2), 140–154. 10.1187/cbe.06-11-0203

Rank, A., & Pool, H. (2014). Writing better writing assignments. *PS: Political Science & Politics*, 47(3), 675–681. 10.1017/S1049096514000821

Ross, D., Loeffler, K., Schipper, S., Vandermeer, B., & Allan, G. M. (2013). Do scores on three commonly used measures of critical thinking correlate with academic success of health professions trainees? A systematic review and meta-analysis. *Academic Medicine*, 88(5), 724–734. 10.1097/acm.0b013e31828b0823

Servati, K. (2012). *Prewriting Strategies and Their Effect on Student Writing.* [Master's thesis, St. Hohn Fisher College]. https://fisherpub.sjfc.edu/cgi/viewcontent.cgi?article=1243&context=education_ETD_masters

Sharma, S. (2010). How to become a competent medical writer?. *Perspectives in Clinical Research*, 1(1), 33. https://www.ncbi.nlm.nih.gov/pmc/articles/PMC3149406/pdf/PCR-1-33.pdf

Stephenson, N. S., & Sadler-McKnight, N. P. (2016). Developing critical thinking skills using the science writing heuristic in the chemistry laboratory. *Chemistry Education Research and Practice*, 17(1), 72–79. 10.1039/C5RP00102A

Stepien W., Gallagher S., & Workman D. (1993). Problem-based learning for traditional and interdisciplinary classrooms. *Journal for the Education of the Gifted*, 16(4), 338–357. 10.1177/016235329301600402

Sykes, S., Wills, J., Rowlands, G., & Popple, K. (2013). Understanding critical health literacy: A concept analysis. *BMC Public Health*, 13(1), 1–10. 10.1186/1471-2458-13-150

The National Commission on Writing. (2003). *The neglected "R"*. The College Board. http://www.vantagelearning.com/docs/myaccess/neglectedr.pdf

Terryberry K. (2005). *Writing for the health professions*. Thomson Delmar Learning.

Tiwari, A., Lai, P., So, M., & Yuen, K. (2006). A comparison of the effects of problem-based learning and lecturing on the development of students' critical thinking. *Medical Education*, 40(6), 547–554. 10.1111/j.1365-2929.2006.02481.x

Wilgis, M., & McConnell, J. (2008). Concept mapping: An educational strategy to improve graduate nurses' critical thinking skills during a hospital orientation program. *The Journal of Continuing Education in Nursing*, 39(3), 119–126. 10.3928/00220124-20080301-12

Zarcadoolas, C., Pleasant, A., & Greer, D. S. (2003). Elaborating a definition of health literacy: A commentary. *Journal of Health Communication*, 8(S1), 119–120. 10.1080/713851982

Appendix 1: Sample Paper with Annotations
Special Thanks to Roshaun Lendore

Paragraph #	Student writing	Annotations
1	The proliferation of mosquitoes in tropical climates is well known. A common mosquito (vector) is the Aedes Aegypti specie, which can transmit vector-borne diseases (VBDs) such as Zika virus, Chikungunya, and dengue fever to humans (Powell et al., 2018). In Grenada, the Aedes Aegypti mosquito was responsible for outbreaks of Chikungunya fever in 2014 (Macpherson et al, 2016), and Zika virus in 2016	This student decided to develop a proposal that addresses the problem of mosquitos in Carriacou because they can transmit vector-borne diseases. When students engage in the process of selecting an issue, they must practice the critical thinking sub-skill **categorization** because they must determine if their issues fall under at least 2 of the 3 domains of One Health.

(Continued)

Paragraph #	Student writing	Annotations
	(Brenciaglia et al., 2018). Furthermore, the mosquito population in Grenada's second-largest island, Carriacou, poses major challenges for residents (Patterson, 2014).	
	Vector control refers to measures to reduce vector proliferation that target the immature or adult stages of the mosquito, categorized as chemical, environmental, or biological control methods (McCall et al., 2009, 2009). Vector control practices prevent VBD transmission by reducing contact between the vector and humans (Wilson et al., 2020). According to a study by Brenciaglia et al. (2018) which analyzed Grenada's response to the 2016 Zika virus outbreak, primarily environmental and chemical control methods are used locally. This study concluded that the vector control measures employed in Grenada, have minimal effect on limiting VBD transmission, and thus recommended that "new and novel approaches to vector control" be used to prevent future VBD outbreaks. A proposal is therefore made for the local Vector Control Unit (VCU) to lay the groundwork for introducing Wolbachia-infected mosquitoes in Carriacou, in collaboration with the WHO/World Mosquito Program (WMP) and the World Health Organization Special Programme in Research and Training in Tropical Diseases (WHO/TDR), with funding from the US Agency for International Development (USAID).	By describing the study conducted by Brenciaglia et al. (2018), this student is both **clarifying meaning** for the reader and **decoding the significance**. They show their ability to **clarify meaning** by paraphrasing the results of the study. They are **decoding significance** by demonstrating how the introduction of Wolbachia-infected mosquitoes in Carriacou will help to limit VBD.

(Continued)

Paragraph #	Student writing	Annotations
2	Current chemical vector control methods used locally are suboptimal. Aerial spray pesticide, commonly referred to as fogging is the major mosquito control method used in Carriacou (Government of Grenada, 2020). However, continuous fogging has been linked to increased resistance of mosquitoes, and an eventually reduced efficacy of fogging measures (Kasai et al, 2014). Furthermore, one of the chemicals used in local fogging practices, Permethrin (Now Grenada, 2015), potentially endangers bees, which play an important role in the local ecosystem (Henry et al., 2012).	In this excerpt, the student is exhibiting the sub-skill **examining ideas** because they are identifying and explaining the various issues associated with fogging for mosquito control. In addition to this, it is evident that here, and throughout the paper, this student is **assessing claims** by using evidence from credible sources to support their proposal. Another critical thinking sub-skill displayed here, and throughout the paper, is **stating results**. This student exhibits this sub-skill by effectively articulating their reasoning.
	While implementation of Wolbachia-infected mosquitoes into the environment would not eliminate the need for current environmental control methods, it would be a valuable tool to augment these. The shortcomings of currently utilized chemical vector control methods illustrate the need for exploring viable alternatives such as biological control methods.	Here we can see the student is showcasing the sub-skill **conjecturing alternatives** as they are providing an alternative to fogging, which is the main method used to control the mosquito population in Carriacou. Here they suggest releasing Wolbachia-infected mosquitos to use in addition to fogging to address the issue.
3	There are concerns regarding the efficacy of this control method in lessening VBD transmission risk, without itself creating further health risks. In an investigation conducted in Cairns, Northern Australia, common concerns among residents pertained to the ability of the Wolbachia bacteria to be transferred to or affect humans, the soil, and other organisms (Popovici, 2010). However, these concerns are unsupported, since the evidence suggests that the risks	This student wanted to provide support for their solution to use Wolbachia-infected mosquitos and this excerpt highlights this student's ability to **query evidence** because they needed to provide evidence to support their claim. Here they provide strong evidence showing that Wolbachia-infected mosquitos do not pose a significant risk to human or environmental health. In doing this, they are also **drawing conclusions** and **presenting**

(Continued)

Paragraph #	*Student writing*	*Annotations*
	posed by introducing Wolbachia mosquitoes into the environment are minimal. Wolbachia have never been identified in humans or other mammals. Furthermore, there is no evidence that bites from Wolbachia-infected mosquitoes, or ingestion of food products with their residues are harmful to humans (Popovici, 2010).	**arguments** by supporting their proposal with sound reasons as one of the best alternatives.
	Biological control of Aedes Aegypti mosquitoes using Wolbachia-infected mosquitoes has been proven effective. A study by McMeniman et al. (2009) found that Wolbachia-infected mosquitoes reduce the lifespan of Aedes Aegypti mosquitoes by up to 50% and is maternally transmitted to 100% of their offspring. Additionally, while not widespread, Wolbachia-infected mosquito introduction has been successful in places such as Yogyakarta, Indonesia, as well as Mourilyan and South Johnstone in North Queensland, Australia (McMeniman et al., 2009). Despite some perceived risks, the evidence strongly suggests that Wolbachia is a safe and effective control method, as seen in its measured success in different countries. Due to similarities in climate, it may be deduced that comparable results can be obtained in Carriacou.	In this excerpt we can see this student is using a few critical thinking sub-skills. They are **justifying procedures** as they are providing evidence and reasoning to justify why using Wolbachia-infected mosquitoes can help address the problem in Carricacou because it has been effective in other areas. Again as in the last paragraph they are **presenting arguments** because their justification provides more reasoning in support of their proposed solution. Lastly, as with many other parts of this paper, this student is **clarifying meaning** because they are paraphrasing results from research.
4	The first step in the proposal is to conduct community engagement with relevant stakeholders. Community engagement is essential for introducing novel vector control methods such as Wolbachia mosquitoes (Liew, 2021). Prevailing evidence	In the first step of their proposal, this student continues to showcase the critical thinking subs-skills they have in previous parts of the paper. Students are required to justify each of their steps and in order to do so they must **query evidence** by finding support for this

(Continued)

Paragraph #	Student writing	Annotations
	emphasizes the importance of inclusive public engagement and consultation when implementing such a proposal (Subramaniam et al. 2012; McNaughton & Duong, 2014). The VCU in conjunction with experts from the World Mosquito Program would host community meetings in villages across the island with residents and other stakeholders including business owners. This is geared towards: a) establishing the need for this control method based on the history of VBDs on the island, and b) educating the public about the efficacy of Wolbachia mosquito control by illustrating its success elsewhere. When initiating any program in a community, its acceptance by stakeholders is paramount since their actions or inactions may either improve or hinder the project's success. Community acceptance upon completing this step increases the probability of the project's success, thus allowing the procession to the next stage of the proposal.	justification. In doing this they are also **justifying procedures** by providing this evidence in support of this step. This is also linked to **presenting arguments** as all this exhibits this student's ability to provide reasons in support of their stance that this is an appropriate first step to tackle this problem.
5	The second step is to build local capacity for the release of the Wolbachia-infected mosquitoes. The WHO/TDR aims to strengthen developing countries' capacity to deploy genetically modified vectors such as Wolbachia, and thus has funded Regional Training Centers in different parts of the world including Colombia, Latin America to train and prepare public health workers in the knowledge and experience necessary for the implementation of biosafety and	The critical thinking sub-skills shown in the next two steps of the proposal mirror those in the first step and are not elaborated on here.

(*Continued*)

Paragraph #	Student writing	Annotations
	regulatory principles (Beech et al., 2009). The novelty of this control method necessitates training of officers in the local VCU in techniques for the safe and efficient deployment of the mosquitoes. The WHO/TDR Regional Training Center in Colombia will assist in this training by sending trainers to Carriacou. Additionally, all the materials necessary for the subsequent step would be procured and imported, including storage units, equipment for mosquito deployment, personal protective equipment. While the cost is not yet determined, budgetary planning is key in launching a funding request, and thus must be first completed before full proceeding to later steps. The funding for these materials would be sought from the USAID. The successful implementation of the proposal requires the technical competency of the VCU, who must be equipped with the necessary tools for the Wolbachia-mosquito release.	
6	Thirdly, the genetics of the Wolbachia mosquitoes for release would be matched with the local Aedes Aegypti population. Due to geographical isolation and unique environmental conditions, the characteristics of Aedes Aegypti mosquitoes vary in different countries because of changes in their genes over time (Lv et al., 2020). Therefore, backcrossing (matching) the traits of the Wolbachia mosquitoes with those of the Aedes Aegypti population endemic to Carriacou (O'Neill et al., 2018), is necessary to facilitate	

Paragraph #	Student writing	Annotations

their invasion and eventual vector control effects by enhancing their chance of adapting to, and surviving in local conditions (Garcia et al., 2019). Ensuring that the biological makeup of the Wolbachia mosquitoes to be released are matched to the local target mosquito population increases their resilience, and the prospect of an eventually successful release, persistence, and survival of the Wolbachia mosquitoes in Carriacou.

7   This proposal is to complete the foundational work necessary for a successful introduction of Wolbachia bacteria-infected mosquitoes in Carriacou by the VCU in collaboration with the WMP, WHO/DTR and USAID, to reduce local VBD transmission. Despite safety concerns, scientific research has proven that the method is safe and effective. The proposal entails community engagement to sensitize the locals about the method, followed by building the VCU's capacity for implementation. Finally, some of Wolbachia mosquitoes' genes would be matched to that of the local Aedes Aegypti population prior to release. The successful release of these mosquitoes should significantly reduce the Aedes Aegypti mosquito population. This will translate into a decreased incidence of VBDs and an improved quality of life for citizens of Carriacou.

Through the feedback process described in our chapter, this student also exhibited the subskills of **self-examination** and **self-correction**. They had to both reflect on their proposal and identify areas of improvement and then revise their paper to address those areas of weakness.

Appendix 2: References in Student Sample Paper

Beech, C. J., Vasan, S., Quinlan, M. M., Capurro, M. L., Alphey, L., Bayard, V., … & Mumford, J. (2009). Deployment of innovative genetic vector control strategies: Progress on regulatory and biosafety aspects, capacity building and development of best-practice guidance. *Asia Pacific Journal of Molecular Biology and Biotechnology*, 17(3), 75–85.

Brenciaglia, M., Noël, T. P., Fields, P. J., Bidaisee, S., Myers, T. E., Nelson, W. M., … & Macpherson, C. N. (2018). Clinical, serological, and molecular observations from a case series study during the Asian lineage Zika virus outbreak in Grenada during 2016. *Canadian Journal of Infectious Diseases and Medical Microbiology*, 2018.

Garcia, G. D. A., Sylvestre, G., Aguiar, R., da Costa, G. B., Martins, A. J., Lima, J. B. P., … & Maciel-de-Freitas, R. (2019). Matching the genetics of released and local Aedes aegypti populations is critical to assure Wolbachia invasion. *PLoS Neglected Tropical Diseases*, 13(1), e0007023.

Government of Grenada (2020, August 31). Commencement of Fogging- Carriacou and Petite Martinique. https://gov.gd/commencement-fogging-carriacou-petite-martinique

Henry, M., Beguin, M., Requier, F., Rollin, O., Odoux, J. F., Aupinel, P., … & Decourtye, A. (2012). A common pesticide decreases foraging success and survival in honey bees. *Science*, 336(6079), 348–350.

Kasai, S., Komagata, O., Itokawa, K., Shono, T., Ng, L. C., Kobayashi, M., & Tomita, T. (2014). Mechanisms of pyrethroid resistance in the dengue mosquito vector, Aedes aegypti: Target site insensitivity, penetration, and metabolism. *PLoS Neglected Tropical Diseases*, 8(6), e2948.

Liew, C., Soh, L. T., Chen, I., Li, X., Sim, S., & Ng, L. C. (2021). Community engagement for Wolbachia-based Aedes aegypti population suppression for dengue control: The Singapore experience. In Hendrichs, J., Pereira, R., & Vreysen, M. J. B. (Eds.), *Area-wide integrated pest management: Development and field application* (pp. 747–761). CRC Press.

Lv, R. C., Zhu, C. Q., Wang, C. H., Ai, L. L., Lv, H., Zhang, B., … & Tan, W. L. (2020). Genetic diversity and population structure of Aedes aegypti after massive vector control for dengue fever prevention in Yunnan border areas. *Scientific Reports*, 10(1), 12731.

Macpherson, C., Noël, T., Fields, P., Jungkind, D., Yearwood, K., Simmons, M., … & LaBeaud, A. D. (2016). Clinical and serological insights from the Asian lneage Chikungunya outbreak in Grenada, 2014: An observational study. *The American Journal of Tropical Medicine and Hygiene*, 95(4), 890–893.

McMeniman, C. J., Lane, R. V., Cass, B. N., Fong, A. W., Sidhu, M., Wang, Y. F., & O'Neill, S. L. (2009). Stable introduction of a life-shortening Wolbachia infection into the mosquito Aedes aegypti. *Science*, 323(5910), 141–144.

McNaughton, D., & Duong, T. T. H. (2014). Designing a community engagement framework for a new dengue control method: A case study from central Vietnam. *PLoS Neglected Tropical Diseases*, 8(5), e2794.

McCall, P., Lloyd, L., & Nathan, M. B. (2009). Vector management and delivery of vector control services. *Dengue guidelines for diagnosis, treatment, prevention and control*. 3rd ed. The World Health Organization.

Now Grenada (2015, June 23). Mosquito fogging. https://www.nowgrenada.com/2015/06/mosquito-fogging/

O'Neill, S. L., Ryan, P. A., Turley, A. P., Wilson, G., Retzki, K., Iturbe-Ormaetxe, I., ... & Simmons, C. P. (2018). Scaled deployment of Wolbachia to protect the community from dengue and other Aedes transmitted arboviruses [version 2; peer review: 2 approved]. *Gates Open Research*, 2. 10.12688/gatesopenres.12844.3

Patterson, R. (2014, October 14). *Environmental Officer Shocked at Mosquito Population.* https://www.thegrenadainformer.com/carriacou/item/1976-environmental-officer-shocked-at-mosquito-population

Powell, J. R., Gloria-Soria, A., & Kotsakiozi, P. (2018). Recent history of Aedes aegypti: Vector genomics and epidemiology records. *Bioscience*, 68(11), 854–860.

Popovici, J., Moreira, L. A., Poinsignon, A., Iturbe-Ormaetxe, I., McNaughton, D., & O'Neill, S. L. (2010). Assessing key safety concerns of a Wolbachia-based strategy to control dengue transmission by Aedes mosquitoes. *Memorias do Instituto Oswaldo Cruz*, 105, 957–964.

Subramaniam, T. S., Lee, H. L., Ahmad, N. W., & Murad, S. (2012). Genetically modified mosquito: The Malaysian public engagement experience. *Biotechnology Journal*, 7(11), 1323–1327.

Wilson, A. L., Courtenay, O., Kelly-Hope, L. A., Scott, T. W., Takken, W., Torr, S. J., & Lindsay, S. W. (2020). The importance of vector control for the control and elimination of VBDs. *PLoS Neglected Tropical Diseases*, 14(1), e0007831.

World Mosquito Program (2021). Wolbachia method: How it works. https://www.worldmosquitoprogram.org/en/work/wolbachia-method/how-it-works

3

FIRST DO NO HARM: PROMOTING HEALTH LITERACIES THROUGH EMPATHY ADVENTURES IN THE WRITING CLASSROOM AND BEYOND

Allison S. Walker

In the Healthy People 2030 campaign, health literacy is defined as follows: "Health literacy occurs when a society provides accurate health information and services that people can easily find, understand, and use to inform their decisions and actions" (U.S. Department of Health and Human Services). This definition of health literacy improves on prior Healthy People programs by adding "society" into the equation and by explicitly promoting healthy "actions" a literate citizen can take when armed with this knowledge. However, this definition still has shortcomings, and a key element is still missing: empathy.

This new definition was discussed extensively during the public comment period, which occurred between June 3, 2019 and August 5, 2019. Stated most succinctly by Commenter 54, a 20-year health literacy advocate from a clinical background, health literacy must include empathy, which is often expressed through listening and shared understanding:

> I feel that the essence of health literacy is not only to communicate clearly but also listen to those we communicate with. Neither party can achieve these goals alone. I created and continue to use a more functional definition of health literacy. It is "Health literacy happens when providers (or anyone on the giving end of health communication) and patients (anyone on the receiving end) *truly understand one another*" (italics added).

This chapter seeks to build on this comment and others that advocate for greater empathy in our conceptualizations of health literacies. I suggest that by approaching health literacies from Commenter 54's "more functional definition," undergraduate writing instructors can more meaningfully contribute to the holistic goals of health and well-being. Relatedly, I suggest that there is an

DOI: 10.4324/9781003316770-5

important place in health literacies for narrative medicine, a theme that Jarron Slater picks up on in Chapter 4.

The assignments discussed in this chapter have been given in multiple sections (*n* = 141 students) of undergraduate writing courses at High Point University. The courses in which they have been assigned have varied in terms of level (first-year composition, honors junior-level seminar, service learning, general education literature, professional writing) and mode of instruction (face-to-face, hybrid, and online). All of the courses were thematically organized around the principles of narrative medicine, providing a foundation in empathy training for health literacies.

The Science of Empathy

Broadly speaking, empathy is the imaginative act of stepping into the shoes of another person, understanding their feelings and perspectives, and using that understanding to guide our actions. Empathy is a core component of narrative medicine, a clinical practice in the health professions that encourages caregivers to recognize and be moved by illness narratives, attending to the narrative structures and techniques embodied in those stories. By focusing health professionals' attention on their own capacity for empathy, or feeling *with* rather than *for* their patients, narrative medicine practitioners often report more positive mental and physical health outcomes from their patients and lower levels of professional burnout themselves. According to Krznaric (2015), "it is by imagining ourselves in the shoes of others ... that we extend our circle of moral concern, develop our sense of justice, and make the leap from a self-interest to a common-interest frame of thinking" (p. 4). In scholarship, psychologists typically divide empathy into two types: affective and cognitive. Affective empathy allows us to mirror other people's emotions. For example, the yawn contagion, the impulse to yawn when you see someone else yawn, is considered one of our most primitive expressions of empathy. Other examples include infants' abilities to mimic the facial expressions of parents (you stick out your tongue, she sticks out hers) and our collective impulse to laugh if someone else laughs or cry if we see someone else crying. Affective empathy (feeling *with* someone synchronously) is different from sympathy (feeling *for* someone) and compassion. According to Krznaric (2019), compassion "does not involve positive emotional resonance" but does describe actionable behaviors in response to witnessing another person's emotional situation (p. 6).

Recent research in the field of neuroscience has provided concrete evidence of our affective empathy system. In the 1990s, scientists discovered "mirror neurons," neural pathways that light up along the same routes when we see someone experiencing an intense emotion as if we were actually experiencing it ourselves (de Waal, 2019). Mirror neurons help us feel what others are feeling, whether that emotion is positive or negative. More recent research demonstrates a complex neural network or empathy circuit in which mirror neurons are only a part, and present-day neuropsychological research uncovers new intricacies of this empathy circuit regularly (de Waal, 2019).

The second type of empathy is cognitive, or perspective-taking, empathy, and it requires a sophisticated use of our imaginations. For example, if you see a video of someone with COVID-19 on a ventilator in a hospital room alone, with no loved ones by their side and caregivers garbed in PPE from head to toe, you might just feel sorry for that person (sympathy). Or you might try to imagine what it feels like to be that person, struggling to breathe, unable to communicate with loved ones or see the facial expressions of caregivers. You might try to imagine that person's struggles, hopes, and fears, or even try to embody their whole being. What do hospital sheets feel like against feverish skin? Does it feel different to hold someone's hand through a latex glove? According to Krznaric (2019), cognitive empathy is important for at least two reasons. First, cognitive empathy gives us the capacity to respond to the needs of others appropriately, even when they come from different sociocultural backgrounds than our own. Second, "throughout human history, the failure to take the perspective of 'the Other' has been at the root of prejudice, exploitation and violence" (Krznaric, 2019, p. 6).

Studies of neural plasticity, our brain's ability to grow new neural pathways, demonstrate that empathy is yet another way in which our brains develop throughout our lives. Yet, it may become more difficult as we age because those neural pathways become somewhat fossilized through repeated and habitual thought patterns (like prejudice) (de Waal, 2019). Basically, we can learn empathy, build empathy, and enhance our innate empathic tendencies, just like we can learn to play the piano or shoot free throws. We have to practice. Our ability to cognitively empathize is hard-wired in our brains, but we have to activate those pathways regularly to keep them. But how?

Krznaric (2019) argues that we can inculcate our cognitive empathy "by making a conscious effort to focus mindfully on the feelings and experiences of other people and species" (p. 8) through the practice of "experiential adventures," or physical and mental activities one engages in consciously, with an open mind and heart, and as a holistic sensory experience, in order to grow one's capacity for empathy. Some examples he cites include an ongoing Canadian project called the "Roots of Empathy" in which an infant regularly visits an elementary classroom throughout the school year so the students can sit in a circle on the floor around the infant and actively engage in conversation about what that baby is thinking and feeling. Another example is a touring interactive museum exhibit in which participants are guided by a blind person through a darkened space that simulates an apartment and a coffee shop so they can experience what daily life might feel like if they were sightless. He believes activities such as these will not only increase our levels of concern for others, but they will motivate us to take action, shifting our collective mindset from "me" to "we."

In the assignments below, I illustrate a series of empathy adventures that took place in undergraduate writing classrooms at a private liberal arts university located in High Point, North Carolina. For an explicitly programmatic approach to teaching reflection, see Chapter 7, where Yuko Taniguchi and colleagues share insights from their work at the University of Minnesota—Rochester.

Assignment 1: "Parallel Chart" (Charon, 2006)

Synopsis

Create an accurate medical chart for one of the main characters in a course literary text (fiction, nonfiction/memoir, poetry, drama) and then create a "parallel chart" (as defined by Charon, 2006, The Parallel Chart) in the voice of that character's caregiver.

Writing Genres

Reflective writing, medical charting, role-playing

Assignment Overview

In order to understand the context of this assignment, one must first recognize the chronic stress workers in the health professions must face throughout their careers in order to provide effective and empathic care to their patients. Health literacies are a two-way street, and empathic communication is unsustainable if both parties aren't willing to enter the dyad with an acknowledgment of their own vulnerabilities. Charon, a practicing physician, literary scholar, and educator invented this technique in 1993, when she recognized a pervasive gap in medical education:

> I found myself unhappy that my students did not have a routine method with which to consider their patients' experiences of illness or to examine what they themselves undergo when caring for patients. We were very effectively teaching students about biological disease processes, and we were systematically training them to do lumbar punctures and to present cases at attending rounds, but we were not being conscientious in helping them to develop their interior lives as doctors. Nor were we modeling methods of recognizing what patients and families go through at the hands of illness and, indeed, at our own hands in the hospital.
>
> *(Charon, 2006, p. 155)*

To fill this gap, she began training her students to practice reflective writing outside the narrow parameters of the traditional medical chart, the SOAP Notes (subjective, objective, assessment, plan) that record the symptoms of a patient, their vital signs and test results, the doctor's diagnosis, and a proposed course of treatment. Within this narrow frame of medical charting, Charon realized there was no space for the doctor to record an authentic emotional responses to the patient. So, she invented the parallel chart. She describes the parallel charting process to her medical students by telling them:

> Every day you write in the hospital chart about each of your patients. You know exactly what to write there, and the form in which to write it. You write about your patient's current complaints, the results of the physical exam, laboratory findings, opinions of consultants, and the plan. If your patient dying of prostate cancer reminds you of your grandfather, who died of that disease last summer, and each time you go into the patient's room, you weep for your grandfather, you cannot write that in the hospital chart. We will not let you. And yet it has to be written somewhere. You write it in the parallel chart.
>
> *(Charon, 2006, p. 155)*

These are the only instructions she provides. She asks them to write at least one parallel chart entry per week during their third year of medical school, and she reminds them that the parallel chart isn't a diary, support group, or therapy. "Instead, the goals are to enable them to recognize more fully what their patients endure and to examine explicitly their own journeys through medicine" (Charon, 2006, p. 157).

In my own undergraduate writing classrooms, filled with undergraduates on a health professions track, the firsthand experiences of Charon's medical students aren't readily available because my students aren't yet working directly with patients in a clinical setting. Some are pursuing other majors and likely will not. So instead, I ask them to imagine themselves there, as potential caregivers for a patient whose illness narrative the students read together: the autobiographical memoir of Amy Fusselman, called *The pharmacist's mate* (2002), in which the author grapples with the recent death of her father and her own struggles with infertility. In this version of a parallel chart assignment, students practice cognitive empathy by role-playing as a caregiver within Amy's narrative, using Charon's students' parallel chart entries as models for their own creative exploration of this reflective writing genre.

Before crafting the parallel chart in the voice of one of Amy's caregivers, however, students must first fill out a traditional medical chart for the patient. They research the SOAP notes process and construct a traditional medical chart that includes relevant medical information gleaned from the literary text (like the patient's name, symptoms, and prescribed medications) and some creative research to fill in any gaps (like the most likely blood pressure of a pregnant 37-year-old white woman of average height and weight living in New York

City in 2001). Once the students have created the traditional medical chart, they become acutely aware of the gaps in it, the gaps a parallel chart could potentially fill. For example, Amy's memoir depicts her ongoing struggle with grief over the death of her father, yet that fact doesn't fit on a traditional obstetric medical chart. When creating a hypothetical parallel chart in the voice of that obstetrician, many students explore Amy's grief and often connect it to a loss of their own, a personal detail they invent for the role of the obstetrician in order to develop some emotional common ground between Amy and her caregiver.

Reflections

The contrast between the impersonal diction of a medical chart ("SWF denies IVF"), often communicated in medical jargon, shorthand, sentence fragments, and third-person distance, and the intimacy of a first-person reflection from the doctor's perspective ("I want to live like her") is illuminated for the student writers, and they often return to the significance of the parallel chart assignment in their final capstone reflections of the semester ("Why it matters") when commenting on the narrative medicine techniques they intend to carry with them into their careers beyond the classroom. Though they are playing a role as a caregiver, a voice separated from their own personal experiences, many students find their own self-identity creeping into the conversation. A number of students over the years have commented on their own relatives' struggles with infertility and the ways Fusselman's memoir of her own failed attempts at fertility treatment made them feel more connected to their own family member's illness narrative. This assignment allows a safe space for students to explore those connections and thus grow their own capacity for cognitive empathy while also developing health literacies along the way. All of them can benefit from the process of decoding a traditional medical chart, learning how to read all those abbreviations and sentence fragments, and many students have commented on their increased confidence in navigating their own digital medical charts after completing this assignment.

Assignment 2: Musical Medicine Empathy Adventure

Synopsis

If you could give a hypothetical patient from one of our literary texts a playlist to help them heal, what songs would you include and why?

Writing Genres

Reflective writing, role-playing

Assignment Overview

All of us have playlists that we curate as the soundtrack to our daily lives. Maybe you have a road trip playlist, a heartbreak playlist, or a playlist you use to get yourself pumped up before the big game. We intrinsically know that music impacts us on both a physical and an emotional level. We remember lyrics to songs we haven't heard in years, yet we can't remember what we read last night. We increase our pace on the treadmill according to the tempo of the song piped through our earbuds. We tie specific songs to specific memories and emotions, and we relive them each time we hear that song for the rest of our lives. No matter your age, gender, culture, or educational level, it is likely that music plays an important part in your self-identity. This assignment seeks to build on this universal human creative endeavor from a narrative medicine perspective by adopting music as a form of mental health medical treatment.

Prior to this assignment, students are exposed to two literary texts that address the impact of music on the speaker's illness narrative, Sabrina Benhaim's (2017) contemporary poetry collection, *Depression and other magic tricks*, and Jean-Dominique Bauby's (1998) memoir, *The diving bell and the butterfly*. While these texts aren't necessary for the successful implementation of this assignment in an undergraduate writing classroom, I will use them as examples to elucidate the context of this particular assignment. Theoretically, any illness narrative would suffice for this assignment, or it could even be revised to focus on the student as a patient, self-prescribing a playlist to therapeutically address one's own mental health narrative. The goal is cognitive empathy, an intellectual process that encompasses a wide range of source texts and academic curricula, and as such, the academic parameters of the assignment are malleable and can be tailored to fit any undergraduate writing classroom.

Benhaim's poetry collection chronicles her diagnosis of depression and her artistic response to it. Bauby's memoir describes his life before and after a stroke that left him physically paralyzed with "locked-in syndrome," the ability to blink one eye his only form of communication. Both texts address the emotional impact of music on the main character's mental state, and thus they provide an opportunity to examine the potential of music as medicine through the application of narrative medicine close reading techniques. Two musically inspired poetry sequences figure prominently in Benhaim's collection. One alludes to Beyoncé's work ("dear Beyoncé (I)"; "dear Beyoncé (II)") as a means of actualizing a confident feminist approach to love and heartbreak, while the other utilizes a unique poetic form known as found poetry in which the author borrows lyrics from popular songs and selectively reconstructs them into a poem that then takes on new meaning based on the poet's structural and aesthetic choices (2017). Benhaim calls these poems "erasures" and uses bars of blacked-out lyrics to visually depict her struggles against the black bars of depression that threaten to keep her prisoner in her own head (e.g., one poem is titled "better together *a Jack Johnson erasure*").

A class discussion of Benhaim's work through the lens of narrative medicine elicits a depth of analysis not easily captured outside a graduate-level creative writing program. Students point to form and frame, two terms described by Charon's "Close reading" (2006) chapter, when exploring the visual affront of the erasure poem in which all of the lyrics are redacted except for the phrase: "I believe in memories / but there is not enough time" (Benaim, 2017). They then raise questions of temporality and illness time, two more of Charon's terms, as they explore what they perceive as the poet's reasoning for including only these two lines from the song. They discuss what's left in the frame of the poem and what's left out, and then eventually a student, unprompted by the instructor, pulls up the song on their smartphone to address the apparent disconnect between the sound and mood of the song itself and the meaning that underlies the poem. The conversation inevitably turns to questions about whether or not this song and the subsequent black bars of its new poetic form are evidence of Benhaim's progress past a bad relationship and toward emotional healing, or whether they are evidence that she's wallowing in difficult memories from her past and thus stunting her own emotional growth by reliving that memory over and over each time she hears this song.

The point of the discussion is that there is no "right" answer. As readers, we can't truly know Benhaim's poetic intentions unless we ask her directly. But the process of exploring these lines of inquiry allows students to practice complex close reading skills on a theoretical level while also practicing cognitive empathy by stepping into the shoes of Benhaim and attempting to see the world, including the conundrums of an esoteric emotional landscape, through her eyes. Some students then choose to create a playlist for Benhaim as they curate a Musical Medicine Playlist from the perspective of her therapist, seeking to provide musical salve to Benhaim's emotional wounds.

In Bauby's memoir, readers are introduced to many musical allusions, from classical, to jazz, to rock and roll. The most prominent and recognizable one for an audience of college students is the Beatles's "A day in the life," the song that was playing on the radio the day Bauby suffered a stroke that forever altered his world. He returns to the song from his "locked-in" perspective in a later chapter, ironically titled "A day in the life," in which he chronicles the frustrations of his illness and its impact on what used to be considered mundane everyday tasks, like navigating Paris traffic or attending boring editorial staff meetings, tasks that are now wholly out of reach for Bauby (1998).

As with Benhaim's allusions to popular songs, students often find more meaning in Bauby's text when they revisit the Beatles's song, particularly the iconic chord of dissonant symphonic sound that seems emblematic of Bauby's stroke, "in which the whole orchestra reaches a crescendo and holds it until the explosion of the final note. Like a piano crashing down seven floors" (p. 121). If students choose to curate a playlist for Bauby, they inevitably include "A day in the life," though to do so means grappling with difficult questions regarding the drama of meaning, a narrative medicine term from Frank,[18] and Bauby's impending death. Would it be beneficial for Bauby to revisit this song, one he was clearly fond of before his stroke, but which is now forever intertwined in his memory with the drama of genesis (of his illness), another of Frank's (2007) terms? Would he find solace in that familiar yet dissonant chord, or would the song encourage Bauby to dwell on the drama of fear and loss (Frank, 2007), incessantly listing in his mind all the activities he can no longer participate in due to his illness?

To answer these questions, students must enact sophisticated levels of creative thinking, close reading, and analysis to construct a playlist (playable as a multimodal text that includes a one-paragraph explanation of each song choice) that would appeal to the vibrant and sardonic wit of Jean-Dominique Bauby.

Reflections

The Musical Medicine Playlist assignment requires a dexterity of creative thought to bring together two typically disparate realms: the academic and the popular. Students must navigate intertextuality, a Charon (2006) term, in order to curate a playlist that responds to a literary text's main character through an academic lens, while utilizing popular music from the student's own daily life. This degree of synthesis requires students to inhabit both a big picture view of the ethical responsibility incumbent in the use of music as a medical or therapeutic intervention and a detailed, zoomed-in focus on song lyrics, melodic moods, and the singularity of the patient. This intellectual balancing act is frequently required in professional settings yet seldom assessed in academic ones. The inclusion of popular music gives students an in-road into this complex creative thinking process and allows them to engage in cognitive empathy perspective-taking from a place of familiarity. The depth of close reading and sentence-level analysis of both the literary texts and the song lyrics of their chosen playlists enables students to extend their development of health literacies by decoding language and information in order to make informed decisions about mental health.

Assignment 3: Poetry Prescription Empathy Adventure

Synopsis

If you were to prescribe a poem as "medicine" to a hypothetical patient, what poem would you choose and why? The goals of this assignment include creative thinking, as defined through an ability to demonstrate basic narrative medicine competencies, to solve complex problems through the application of role-playing and close reading analysis techniques, to engage in perspective-taking thought processes that enhance one's capacity for cognitive empathy, and, ultimately, to synthesize scholarship, creativity, and real-world health scenarios in order to facilitate healing. As in the previous Musical Medicine Playlist assignment, the Poetry Prescription allows students to continue honing those close reading and sentence-level analytical skills that aid their development of health literacies by engaging with language in its most subtle forms of symbolism and metaphor.

Writing Genres

Reflective writing, role-playing

Assignment Overview

This assignment borrows from the clinical practice of poet and practicing physician Rafael Campo, Director of Literature and Writing Programs at the Humanities Initiative of Harvard Medical School and author of the acclaimed poetry collection, *What the body Told,* (1997) and the academic memoir, *A doctor's black bag of poetry* (2003). Campo (2003) routinely "prescribes" poems to his patients as part of his medical practice and acknowledges that "perhaps the best that poetry can do is to contain, for some of us, our emotions. Perhaps, in this way, it could leave a record, a kind of document that some might cast aside but that others might encounter with relief, and hope, and gratitude" (p.4). While this poetry prescription may not heal the body, it has the capacity to speak beyond the realm of the physical. Campo writes that poetry transformed his own work as a caregiver "from a passive observer, capable only of recasting knowledge of diseases into competent treatment plans, into an active, wise participant in the catholic drama of illness, with the power to heal the soul, if not always the body." He adds, "I could prescribe any of a dozen antibiotics to cure endocarditis, or even a thrombolytic agent to stave off a heart attack; but what I yearned for was the elixir of poetry, which could heal the otherwise untreatable condition of a broken heart."

This assignment asks students to follow in his footsteps by role-playing as caregivers and examining the viability of poems as a treatment for hypothetical patients. In this role-playing scenario, students must choose from one of five selected poems assigned as reading in the course. Then they explore the possibilities of that particular poem as a prescription for two hypothetical patients, one of whom would benefit from this poetry prescription, and another who would not. The poems themselves are analyzed collaboratively within the classroom prior to the completion of this assignment, and the poems are as follows:

- Raymond Carver: "What the doctor said"
- Marie Howe: "What the living do"
- Jane Kenyon: "Let evening come"
- Dorianne Laux: "Aphasia"
- Dylan Thomas: "Do not go gentle into that good night"

While any poem that loosely adheres to the thematic content of illness could be used in this assignment, these particular poems have been chosen because of their relevance to the narrative medicine course curricula and this author's admiration for these poems from an aesthetic perspective. These poems present an array of diverse illness narratives and utilize varied elements of poetic craft and point of view to communicate those narratives to a reader.

To understand how this assignment might work, let's consider a few examples. A patient suffering from a Stage 4 inoperable cancer who has exhausted all means of treatment and stands on the brink of financial ruin as a result of the exorbitant costs of those failed interventions would probably not benefit from the poetic pleas of Dylan Thomas (1952, 1953) to "rage, rage against the dying of the light." Pushing such a patient to keep fighting a losing battle would result in more suffering for that patient and their family. However, a young patient who is struggling to get off a ventilator as a result of COVID-19 might respond more appropriately, for the idea that she should not "go gentle into that good night" could give her the emotional strength needed to continue fighting and finally win her battle against the virus and breathe again on her own.

In contrast, a poem by Jane Kenyon (2005) that encourages her to "Let the wind die down. Let the shed / go black inside. Let evening come," could have the opposite effect, encouraging, instead, her submission to the inevitability of death. However, the patient with Stage 4 cancer might find this poem oddly comforting, particularly its conclusion: "Let it come as it will, and don't / be afraid. God does not leave us / comfortless, so let evening come."

As Campo (2003) says, "we come to poetry, I think, because we are silenced in many ways. In biomedicine, we're so good at appropriating the narrative—the biopsy report, the CT count, the potassium level." Receiving poetry as a therapeutic technique "gives patients an opportunity to say, this is *my* cancer, this is *my* HIV. It's not a generic, what you see on the mammogram or how many lymph nodes are positive—I'm an individual" (p. 3). A poem can offer that patient a prescription to heal the soul, and though that patient may not be inclined to write poetry herself, she may yet be inspired to consume its passion, its magic, and its healing power and make it her own.

Reflections

By exploring the hidden significance of language as not only a conveyor of information but a touchstone for the fragility of the human condition, students gain a deeper understanding of the social factors and situational context of health literacies. To assess this assignment, I use an adaptation of the American Association of Colleges and Universities VALUE Rubric for Creative Thinking, which can be viewed on their website.

Assignment 4: Why Empathy Matters Reflection

Synopsis

Reflect on your evolution as a student in this course. Why does empathy matter, and how might you apply what you learned about narrative medicine to your future career and your own illness narratives?

Writing Genres

Reflective writing, role-playing

Assignment Overview

The final reflective writing assignment of the course doesn't require much explanation. Instructors across all disciplines often assign a reflective writing prompt as a way to bring the course to a close. These reflections are designed to encourage metacognition, and successful attempts will demonstrate a students' mastery of the course learning objectives as they describe the ways in which one confronted learning challenges and overcame intellectual obstacles in pursuit of holistic growth and a final passing grade. This particular final reflection, however, asks students to take this metacognitive work one step further by applying what was learned in the course to the student's own real world professional future and life as a mortal human being. To achieve this transfer of knowledge, students must explore their own work across texts and contexts, within and beyond disciplinary boundaries, and evaluate empathy as a means of cultivating "outrospection," or the ability to look outward at the world and others inhabiting it in order to gain introspective insight into our own consciousness (Krznaric, 2014). Finally, successful reflections will embody both an increased awareness of one's own societal health literacies and reflective empathy, as students reflect on their ability to feel with others and interpret illness narratives through the lens of narrative medicine in order to uncover hidden significance within the relationships between caregivers, the ill, and those who bear witness.

Having stepped into the shoes of others through various role-playing assignments throughout the semester, the final reflection gives students an opportunity to confidently inhabit their own distinct voices, reflecting on their own personal goals as future health professionals and empowering them to embrace their own health literacies as a patient, a professional, a caregiver and a witness. Students instinctively bring the conversation full circle, often returning to the illness narrative they shared in the first reflective writing assignment in order to re-see those narratives again from their evolved perspective. To assess this assignment, I use an adaptation of the American Association of Colleges and Universities' VALUE Rubric for Reflection.

Discussion

While I have primarily assessed the effectiveness of these assignments through qualitative data derived from the students' own writing, some compelling quantitative data also exists. In a one-question survey, undergraduates ($n = 141$) in my professional writing courses rated their agreement with following statement, "Bedside manner: You've either got it, or you don't." Their ratings used a 5-point Likert scale from *strongly agree* to *strongly disagree*. At the beginning of the semester, the majority of students (66.67%) responded that they either *strongly agreed* or *agreed* with the statement about bedside manner. This indicates that the majority of incoming students viewed bedside manner, a term often used as shorthand for empathy in the healthcare settings, as a fixed trait that one inherits from birth.

By the end of the semester, however, those trends reversed drastically, with an overwhelming majority (73.33%) of respondents indicating that they either *strongly disagreed* or *disagreed* with the same statement. This implies that those students' views of bedside manners were influenced by the course content and empathy training completed during the semester. The students thus revised their initial views of bedside manner/empathy and now saw it in a new light, as a malleable trait that can be cultivated and ultimately improved with focused training and practice.

These data trends were also strongly supported by the written reflections of the students, which provide additional evidence of empathy's value in the context of health literacies and undergraduate writing.

5 Practical Suggestions for Implementing Empathy Adventures in Your Undergraduate Writing Classroom

Below you will find five ways to bring empathy into your classroom, which can help students cultivate a range of health literacies. These principles are infinitely adaptable to any range of course curricula and diverse student populations.

Explicitly define empathy: feeling *with*, not *for;* this includes a practical explanation of the difference between affective and cognitive empathy, so students understand the goal of empathy training resides in the cognitive, perspective-taking exercise of empathy.

Emphasize the biological basis of empathy: totally, 98% of human beings are born with the capacity for empathy in the mirror neuron pathways of our brains; while that neural network is innate (nature), it takes practice to further develop and refine it (nurture) and that's exactly what empathy adventures are designed to do.

Expose students to texts that evoke emotion: numerous examples are given in this chapter, but any text will do, as long as it contains an emotionally resonant first-person account of an individual's struggle; "text" also doesn't have to be a purely written form and can include films, songs, images, and podcasts such as the Empathy Museum podcast series; students should be given a "content warning" before tackling any emotionally challenging text.

Utilize outrospection and reflective writing as self-care strategies: remind students that these are tools that require use to keep them sharp; when students internalize outrospective reflection in their daily lives, rather than seeing the process as an isolated academic tactic for one semester in one class, the work then becomes a self-care strategy that instills lifelong empathic growth and supports their own mental health and emotional wellbeing. Encourage students to keep journals, to remain intellectually curious about others, and to seek out experiences that allow them to learn more about themselves by considering another person's perspective. It's also important to remind them that empathy is not endorsement. You don't have to agree with someone to connect with them.

Model empathy every day: Everhart et al. (2016) confirm that guided experiential and reflective learning activities create scaffolding for the development of empathy, enabling students to develop empathic skills beyond what they could reach on their own. If students see you embodying the very empathy you're asking them to cultivate, they will respond in kind. All of the empathy adventures described in this chapter have been attempted by the author. Empathy is a two-way street. For example, since COVID hit in the spring of 2020, the author has added a mental health statement to her syllabi, attended bereavement training so she can better support students who have lost a loved one, and relaxed her attendance and late work policies to account for the mental health concerns of her students.

Empathy provides all of us an opportunity for lifelong learning. It is recognized as a vital life skill in the *Framework for twenty-first century civic learning and democratic engagement* (National Task Force, 2012, p.4), enabling us to honor our shared humanity and engage with the most pressing moral questions of our time. It is a bedrock of college education, of writing instruction, and of health literacies in our pluralistic, deeply interconnected worlds.

References

Bauby, J.-D., & Leggatt, J. (1998). *The diving bell and the butterfly: A memoir of life in death.* Knopf Doubleday.

Benaim, S. (2017). *Depression and other magic tricks.* Button Poetry.

Brown, B. (2010, June). *The power of vulnerability.* [Video]. TEDx. https://www.ted.com/talks/brene_brown_the_power_of_vulnerability?language=en

Campbell L. (2017). The rhetoric of health and medicine as a "teaching subject": Lessons from the medical humanities and simulation pedagogy. *Technical Communication Quarterly*, 27(1), 7–20. doi:10.1080/10572252.2018.1401348

Campo, R. (2003). *The healing art: A doctor's black bag of poetry.* W.W. Norton.

Campo, R. (1997). *What the body told*. Duke University Press.

Carver, R. (1996). What the doctor said. Best Poems. https://www.best-poems.net/raymond_carver/what_the_doctor_said.html

Charon, R. (2006). Close reading. In: *Narrative medicine: Honoring the stories of illness*. Oxford University Press.

Charon R. (2011, Nov.). Honoring the stories of illness. [Video]. TEDx. https://www.youtube.com/watch?v=24kHX2HtU3o

Charon, R. (2006). Narrative features of medicine. In: *Narrative medicine: Honoring the stories of illness*. Oxford University Press.

Charon, R. (2006). The parallel chart. In: *Narrative medicine: Honoring the stories of illness*. Oxford University Press.

Department of Economic and Social Affairs: Disability. (2006). *Convention on the Rights of Persons with Disabilities (CRPD)*. United Nations. un.org. https://www.un.org/development/desa/disabilities/convention-on-the-rights-of-persons-with-disabilities.html

Everhart, R., Elliot, K., & Pelco, L. (2016). *Empathy activators: Teaching tools for enhancing empathy development in service-learning classes*. Virginia Commonwealth University (VCU) Scholars Compass.

Frank, A. W. (2007). Five dramas of illness. *Perspectives in Biology and Medicine*, 50(3), 379–394. doi:10.1353/pbm.2007.0027

Frank, A. W. (2013). *The Wounded storyteller: Body, illness, and ethics*. The University of Chicago Press.

Fusselman, A. (2002). *The pharmacist's mate*. Penguin Books.

Howe, M. (1998). What the living do. Academy of American Poets. poets.org. https://poets.org/poem/what-living-do

Kenyon, J. (2005). Let evening come. Poetry Foundation. Poetryfoundation.org. https://www.poetryfoundation.org/poems/46431/let-evening-come

Kenzie D., & McCall, M. (2017). Teaching writing for the health professions: Disciplinary intersections and pedagogical practice. *Technical Communication Quarterly*, 27(1), 64–79. doi:10.1080/10572252.2017.1402573

Konrath, S. H., O'Brien, E. H., & Hsing, C. (2011, May). Changes in dispositional empathy in American college students over time: A meta-analysis. *Personality and Social Psychology Review*, 15(2), 180–198. doi: 10.1177/1088868310377395

Krznaric, R. (2014). *Empathy: A handbook for revolution*. Penguin Random House.

Krznaric, R. (2014, Jan.). TED Talk: How to start an empathy revolution. [Video]. TEDx. https://www.youtube.com/watch?v=RT5X6NIJR88

Krznaric, R. (2015, March). *The empathy effect: How empathy drives common values, social justice, and environmental action*. Friends of the Earth. Available at: https://policy.friendsoftheearth.uk/sites/default/files/documents/2019-02/empathy-effect.pdf

Laux, D. (2010). Aphasia, Broadsided Press. https://broadsidedpress.org/broadsides/aphasia/

National Task Force on Civic Learning and Democratic Engagement. (2012). *A crucible moment: College learning and democracy's future*. Washington, D.C.: American Association of Colleges and Universities.

Pennebaker J. (1997). *Opening up: The healing power of confiding in others*. The Guilford Press.

Plath, S. (1963). *The bell jar*. Heineman.

Reiss, H. (2013, Dec.). The power of empathy. [Video]. TEDx. YouTube. https://www.youtube.com/watch?v=baHrcC8B4WM

Rodriguez, J. E., Welch, T. J., & Edwards, J. C. (2012). Impact of a creative arts journal on a medical school community: A qualitative study. *Journal of Poetry Therapy*, 25(4), 197–204.

Shem, S. (1978) *The house of God*. Richard Marek Publishers.

Span, P. (2019). Ageism: A 'prevalent and insidious' health threat. *The New York Times*. https://www.nytimes.com/2019/04/26/health/ageism-elderly-health.html

Spreng, R. N., McKinnon, M. C., Mar, R. A., & Levine, B. (2009). The Toronto empathy questionnaire: Scale development and initial validation of a factor-analytic solution to multiple empathy measures. *Journal of Personality Assessment*, 91(1), 62–71. doi:10.1080/00223890802484381

Study of Medical Student, Resident, and Physician Suicide. (2019). American Medical Association. https://www.ama-assn.org/system/files/2019-07/a19-cme-6.pdf

Thomas, D. (1952, 1953). Do not go gentle into that good night. poets.org. https://poets.org/poem/do-not-go-gentle-good-night

Tyson P. (2001, March 27). *The Hippocratic Oath Today*. PBS. https://www.pbs.org/wgbh/nova/article/hippocratic-oath-today/

U.S. Department of Health and Human Services. (2021, August 4). *Health Literacy in Healthy People 2030*. health.gov https://health.gov/our-work/national-health-initiatives/healthy-people/healthy-people-2030/health-literacy-healthy-people-2030

Varnum, M. E. W., Blais, C., Hampton, R. S., & Brewer, G. A. (2015). Social class affects neural empathic responses. *Culture and Brain*, 3(2), 122–130. doi:10.1007/s40167-015-0031-2

Verghese, A. A doctor's touch. [Video]. TED.com. https://www.ted.com/talks/abraham_verghese_a_doctor_s_touch

Waal, F.B.M. de. (2019). *The age of empathy: Nature's lessons for a kinder society*. Souvenir Press.

4

RHETORICAL AESTHETICS AND HEALTH LITERACIES

Jarron Slater

Teaching literature – including rhetoric – should be a key element of under-graduate writing courses focused on health literacies. Building on Allison Walker's discussions in the previous chapter, I argue that literature-as-rhetoric can provide the groundwork for writing more technical documents because it can help to emphasize the human element – the people – involved in health literacies. Literature-as-rhetoric, a subset of rhetorical aesthetics, emphasizes the importance of heartfelt communication, unity between patient and physician, and humanity.

In this chapter, I discuss a writing course I redesigned for students at a small liberal arts university in the Midwest who were interested in careers in health sciences, health care leadership, and nursing. I redesigned the course to include a health humanities and narrative medicine component, based on rhetorical aesthetics, that focuses on individuals and prepares students to write in more technical genres.

Because literacy comprises not just receiving, reading, understanding, and obtaining information but also the capacity to feel, experience, create, and or-ganize information in such a way that people can obtain, understand, and act on it, my discussion of rhetorical aesthetics augments definitions of health literacies to include the essential feelings and experiential aspects of individuals. A rheto-rical aesthetic in the health literacies classroom reveals that health literacies are best understood when they are not separated from emotional and other huma-nistic aspects of health but are expanded to include the unquantifiable, heartfelt understanding of human beings, including oneself. There is no chasm between argument and literature, message and art, rhetoric and aesthetics, but these things overlap, even if they are not the same. Although processes and procedures are important, people are even more important; people matter more than things or even concepts, and they are the essence of why we do what we do.

DOI: 10.4324/9781003316770-6

While literacy certainly includes the capacity of individuals to receive, read, understand, obtain, and act on information, literacy also includes much more: when individuals become increasingly literate, and when we provide others with opportunities to become increasingly literate, we participate in the formation and transformation of identity. Thus, health literacies have the potential to change – to transform – individuals' identities.

I examine this process of identity transformation through the lens of rhetorical aesthetics to argue that a pedagogy of health literacies based on rhetorical aesthetics can improve health literacies. Rhetorical aesthetics comprises an overlap between information management and artistic experience; includes producing texts as well as accessing, understanding, and using them; and emphasizes the transformation of people's identities over concepts or theories. In sum, and as an additional voice to Karen Groller's argument in Chapter 1, I illustrate that undergraduate students who study health literacies should know not just how health information is accessed, understood, and used but also how it is produced. Successfully producing health information involves deep and heartfelt listening to individuals. And that deep and heartfelt listening can be aided by studying health humanities and narrative medicine, both of which have roots in rhetorical aesthetics.

Rhetorical Aesthetics and Health Literacies

Health literacies relate to rhetorical aesthetics because both involve influence through words and symbols to invite others to believe, understand, and act. Rhetorical aesthetics even provides a groundwork that makes health literacies possible. Rhetorical aesthetics helps us to focus on individuals and to see that they are more important than materials and methods. In this section, I provide working definitions of both "rhetoric" and "aesthetics." I show that rhetorical aesthetics enables people to act together by providing them with experiences that shape a collective identity. As acting together fosters an identity transformation for all involved, it naturally leads to a pedagogy that emphasizes people over and above – but without neglecting – concepts, theories, systems, and processes. Understanding the close relationship between rhetoric and aesthetics is important because it can support a pedagogy that rehumanizes and equalizes by inviting action, valorizing genuine listening and empathy, and promoting shared experience.

Health Literacies Through Rhetoric, Identification, and Aesthetics

Rhetoric is often associated with persuasion, argumentation, and influence, as well as with composing for specific audiences. As such, rhetoric includes the use of words and symbols to invite people to identify with one another and thereby cooperate with one another. So, one useful way to understand rhetoric in general – and health literacies in particular – is through the rhetorical aesthetic concept of identification.

Identification, whether in health literacies or in other domains, occurs when people believe that their interests are joined (Burke, 1969). Identification is possible when people speak the same language – and "language" can refer to "speech, gesture, tonality, order, image, attitude, idea," and so on (Burke, 1969, p. 55). Individuals who identify with one another can be understood as being of the same substance, or consubstantial, without denying their distinctness. Those who consubstantially identify are said to be "*acting-together*" and "have common sensations, concepts, images, ideas, [and] attitudes" (Burke, 1969, p. 21; emphasis in original). As such, identification can be a way of understanding empathy (Clark, 2015). Of course, this identification, this empathy, is never total, since people always remain separate entities, but peoples' division is also never total, given human beings' biologic and symbolic similarities (Burke 1931/1968, 78–79; Burke, 1966). Thus, while people who identify become "consubstantial," the term is also inherently – and necessarily – ambiguous because people who identify are both the same in some ways and different in others.

The rhetorical aesthetic concept of identification also provides an understanding of rhetoric's relationship to the aesthetic. Rhetoric is traditionally associated with persuasion and argumentation and the aesthetic with art, story, and experience. Rhetorical aesthetics sees the common ground between art and argument, story and message, persuasion and experience. Rhetoric, in its most effective manifestations, provides people with an aesthetic experience that influences, forms, and can even change identity. The concept of identification is broader than persuasion because identification includes "partially 'unconscious' factor[s]" in appeal (Burke, 1967, p. 63), factors that include peoples' innate capacities to experience, be interested in, and be attracted by the aesthetic. People are drawn to the charm and intrigue of beauty, art, and the sensori-emotional, each of which can lead people to *want* to be persuaded or to experience fulfillment. And this desire to be persuaded or to experience fulfillment, whether intrinsic, intentional, or unintentional, ultimately happens through attitudes of collaborative expectancy associated with the thing that people find attractive (see Slater, 2018).

The rhetorical aesthetic concept of identification helps those who study, practice, and teach health literacies because identification assumes that only what people persuade themselves to do and to become matters. Identification implies self-persuasion; ultimately, people are their own audiences (Burke, 1969). And self-persuasion, whether spontaneous, intuitive, implicit, or unconscious, happens through identification (Burke, 1966) and people's choices to identify. Other people's voices can be effective only if they speak the language of a person's inner voice (Burke, 1969). People who study, practice, and teach health literacies can implement practices that help undergraduate students to persuade themselves by speaking the language of a person's inner voice. Doing so necessitates and enables a focus on people – who they are, what they care about, and why they do the things they do.

Rhetorical Aesthetics and Health Literacies Pedagogy

The difference between aesthetics and the aesthetic is the difference between the branch of philosophy that deals with the study of the beautiful (aesthetics) and the experience that art and the beautiful can provide (the aesthetic). Rhetoric has held common ground with aesthetics since its beginning (Walker, 2000). The word "aesthetic" is often associated with artistic productions and expressions, but it also includes the embodied experiences of both artist and audience. As such, aesthetic expression and aesthetics, also called poetics, can refer more to an effect or an experience rather than a text or a genre (Clark, 2015). The aesthetic breaks down barriers, is the most universal form of language, and is the most effective form of communication (see Dewey, 1934). Aesthetic works can potentially influence, affect, and move a wide variety of people from a wide variety of cultures. For teachers of undergraduate writing, I offer brief background information about rhetorical aesthetics, which may at first seem like an unfamiliar concept.

Just as rhetoric has been associated with aesthetics since its beginning, rhetoric is also inseparable from pedagogy (Graff & Leff, 2005; Heath, 2017). As such, it involves invitations to both discover and form identity. While ancient teachers discuss rhetoric in terms of teaching, delighting, and moving (Cicero, 2001; Quintilian, 2001), they also hinted, and contemporary teachers of rhetoric and literacy know, that these roles are intertwined. Certainly our primary goal as teachers is to teach, but even as we do so, we also understand that delighting and moving are essential components of instruction because students who are engaged, interested, and having fun also remember more, learn quicker, and understand better. In health literacies and beyond, learning and teaching is an aesthetic process as much as a rhetorical one.

The aesthetic also performs the rhetorical work of transforming identity. A person's identity depends on the various identifications that the person acknowledges, defines, assumes, believes, and constructs. These identifications can come from communities, congregations, companies, institutions, friends, and other groups with which a person interacts, associates, communes, serves, uses, cooperates, or, in a word, identifies. Identity is not entirely private or individual, nor can it ever be fully public or universal. In some sense, identity is constantly in flux.

While discussions of the aesthetic usually emphasize making, expressing, or producing a work of art, a scholar of rhetorical aesthetics Gregory Clark (2004) has stated that the aesthetic also provides "considerable rhetorical power": when the aesthetic instantiates experience into symbols that others can appreciate, understand, and experience, its rhetorical power also transforms the identities of those who experience it (p. 52). As teachers of students who are actively developing health literacies – and who will help others become more health literate – we are not just interested in getting people to find, understand, use, make, produce, or even persuade; we, too, are involved in the work of transforming identities.

A person's identity can rest on that person's perception of what it means to be educated, but to be educated involves a transformation of identity (see Westover, 2018). James Berlin (1982) famously stated that when we teach writing, we are not just providing useful training or teaching an important skill but "are teaching a way of experiencing the world, a way of ordering and making sense of it." Berlin continued, "Subtly informing our statements about invention, arrangement, and even style are assumptions about the nature of reality" (p. 776). Here, Berlin is hinting at the potential for educational rhetoric to transform identities. The assumptions we make as teachers can have a powerful, but not always conscious, influence on our students, an influence that can in turn affect students' perceptions of themselves.

The recurring rhetorical work of identity transformation via the aesthetic is evidence that rhetoric has a much broader application and includes much richer implications than is sometimes attributed to it. To divide literature from writing, and rhetoric from aesthetics, is a fake polarity (Booth, 1981). And to pretend that there is a polarity between the two neglects one of the most important parts of persuasion. If Plato's Gorgias, who placed persuasion over knowledge, is still relevant today, one thing that he may teach is that knowing how to help someone is often not enough; helping someone also involves persuading them to act – and it is for this reason that he believed that a rhetorician could more effectively persuade a patient than a physician (see Plato, 2009).

This persuasion happens most effectively when speaker/writer and audience identify with one another, when both parties believe and understand that their interests are joined, and when they see themselves as two parts of one whole – a whole that transcends the identities of the individuals without collapsing them, allowing both to pursue a higher and more whole identity than either could achieve alone. This kind of identification involves a felt aesthetic experience that cannot quite be measured or reported yet nevertheless has a strong influence. It is, after all, what we call rhetoric.

What this means is that we need to include rhetoric and aesthetics as part of our health literacies instruction. A health literacies pedagogy based on a rhetorical aesthetic provides the groundwork for writing more technical documents because it emphasizes communication, consubstantiality between patient and care worker, and, above all, humanity. In addition, because a rhetorical aesthetic calls attention to or at least hints at the ineffable, the indefinable, the messiness, and the unmeasurable aspects of life, becoming acquainted with it helps writers to value the clarity required for writing technical documents. As Campbell (2018) has argued, experts in rhetoric, health humanities, and narrative medicine all have much to learn from one another. Meanwhile, an understanding of rhetoric's bond with aesthetics supports a pedagogy that rehumanizes and equalizes because it invites action, promotes shared experience, and valorizes genuine listening and empathy – three keys to effective health literacies. For a more in-depth discussion of our need to include empathy in our discussions – and our definitions – of health literacies, please see Walker's discussion of it in the previous chapter. In short, rhetorical aesthetics describes the power, capacity, and potential that peoples' experiences with art and the beautiful have to persuade, influence, and even transform the identities of people.

In the following sections, I describe how an undergraduate writing course taught from the perspective of rhetorical aesthetics can emphasize people by inviting action, promoting shared experience, and valorizing genuine listening and empathy. Based on student feedback, this course has been valuable for students' personal, academic, and professional development of health literacies.

Rhetorical Aesthetics, Production, and the Self

As rhetorical aesthetics helps us focus on forming and transforming identity, a pedagogy informed by rhetorical aesthetics emphasizes the importance of individuals through listening to and understanding the experiences of the self and others. In this and the following section, I discuss the following class exercises that invite action, promote shared experiences, and valorize genuine listening and empathy that help students understand this concept: writing in a journal by hand, writing a paper in first person that invited them to discover course concepts for themselves, taking a midterm exam, and writing a *pathography*, or a first-person narrative about illness. Each of these tasks invites action, promotes shared experiences, and valorizes genuine listening and empathy.

Writing by Hand

Students chat until the class begins. I am writing a question on the whiteboard for students to consider. These questions are generally reflective, inviting introspection and thoughtful application of concepts to students' own lives. After prefacing the question, I invite students to write by hand in a journal, a small, simple notebook. While writing by hand may seem somewhat unfashionable these days, it is an embodied experience that helps writers to think more deliberately about the words that they use. Writers who write by hand must physically press down on a piece of paper with a writing instrument and trace each letter of each word by moving their palm, fingers, wrist, and arm. Compared to typing, writing by hand invites writers to use more of their bodies in the act of writing. It also takes longer than typing, thus allowing more time for writers to think about the ideas that they are forming with each successive word.

Because writing by hand requires writers to physically craft each letter of each word, writing by hand invites writers to experience the physical act of writing in a more aesthetic way than typing. It reminds the writer of the writer's own embodiedness and hints at the embodiedness of other individuals. It is not a replacement for typing, but it is a useful and important activity that can facilitate learning. Meanwhile, after students write by hand in their journals, they discuss the question and their response with another student, sometimes for as long as seven to ten minutes. While in this chapter I often use the term "students," in class I tend to avoid that term and instead use the more inclusive "class members" because I see all of us together as being on a journey of discovery. There is an important sense in which all class members are "students."

Discovering Course Content for One's Self

Throughout the course, I invite class members to discover for themselves a relationship between the humanities, health, and writing and then articulate their understanding of this relationship and why their understanding of this relationship matters. I extend this invitation because I believe that the aesthetic can perform the rhetorical work of transforming identity and that transforming identity necessarily involves self-discovery. Since the creative act of rhetorical articulation involves the aesthetic act of rendering experience into a symbol (see Clark, 2004), acts of self-discovery – such as writing – prepare students to become the creators that lie at the summit of Bloom's revised taxonomy of educational objectives (see Anderson et al., 2001). And since the aesthetic breaks down barriers, is the most universal form of language, and is the most effective form of communication (Dewey, 1934), providing opportunities for undergraduate students to discover and create works that others can experience and appreciate will help those students learn more about communication, especially in contexts relating to health literacies.

To embark on this discovery, class members study readings such as those from medical and health humanities (Cole et al., 2015) and narrative medicine (Charon, 2006; Charon et al., 2015), a play (Edson, 1999), poetry, short stories (such as Ewald, 1991), a memoir (Brown, 2010; 2016), and several articles (DasGupta, 2008; Mangino, 2014; Sheilds, 2016; and others). As we study these texts together, class members consider, discuss, analyze, and evaluate how texts change, influence, add to, or complicate their understanding of the relationship between the humanities, health, and communication; how these texts converse with one another; what issues are at stake; and who cares – and who should care. Students discuss what they are learning; what attracts or repels them from the study of health and the humanities; what the costs, benefits, strengths, and drawbacks of studying health, the humanities, and writing are; why they chose to study health; the extent to which they have seen a dehumanization or rehumanization of care; how they guard against dehumanizing tendencies; and how they rehumanize their own work. The result of this journey of discovery can be a paper, a multimodal work, or a short presentation.

For this project, students, individually and in groups, practice teaching the rest of the class about a health humanities topic they have studied. Open-ended class time to discuss the topic provides students with the freedom to share their thoughts, feelings, and experiences and to progress without being bound to a formula. It also helps them to learn to clearly articulate their own understanding of the topic to their primary audience: every member of the classroom. Open-ended prompts also challenge students to figure out what they will say (invention/*invenio*), how they will organize it (arrangement/*dispositio*), and how they will say it (style/*elocutio*).

This open-endedness can be challenging for students who are used to receiving a set of rules or instructions to follow precisely. That is why I teach students about storytelling. I explain to students that writing a paper, even a technical paper, is like telling a story (Burke, 1937/1984). The terms are characters. Some terms become friends, others enemies. Some unite, change, or are transformed. Others depart, stay static, or lie dormant. When we write, whatever it is that we write, we are writing a "story" for our readers to listen to, understand, and experience for themselves.

This discovery activity can be understood as a personal narrative of a student's journey through the class readings from the first part of the semester, a narrative in which the student describes something discovered, piece by piece, as they studied the material, presented on it, and discussed it in class. The multimodal project and presentation lead students to their discovery paper. I invite students to use first-person pronouns for their discovery paper, which may seem strange in a class in which they will later be expected to write papers in a more technical style. Writing in first person can be more complicated – and even more nuanced – than opponents of the idea often think, and it can also both motivate students and more effectively engage readers (Paley, 2001). Practicing making claims in first person can prepare writers to write from the third-person point of view because it helps them discover their own voices, which they must do before they can expand that voice by writing in other genres.

Some writers misinterpret writing in the first person as an overly casual style, but that misinterpretation can be corrected early on by teaching students the importance of striking a balance in their writing between being personable and professional, though the fulcrum can move depending on elements of the rhetorical situation, such as the audience, genre, and context. That sweet spot – formal without being bureaucratic, friendly without being casual, authoritative without being condescending – is a balance that writers must attain every day in their professional lives, a balance that leads to effective health literacies.

Literature and stories can also teach what DasGupta (2008) describes as *narrative humility*. "Narrative humility," a more apt term than "cultural competency," does not assume "mastery" of someone else's story but invites practitioners to learn from and be changed by it. The concept of narrative humility also creates the potential for a transformation of identity that includes a both/and perspective rather than an either/or perspective (see also Clark, 2000). Narrative humility can be acquired through the rhetorical aesthetic experience of literature and stories.

Theresa Brown's work is particularly valuable for teaching writing and health literacies from the perspective of rhetorical aesthetics. Brown's background as a registered nurse with a PhD in English literature is instructive. She has published articles for a variety of audiences and purposes, and in a variety of contexts and styles such as in scholarly journals, in the *New York Times*, and in more popular venues for public audiences. Studying her work helps reinforce the need for attendance to the rhetorical situation. In her memoir *The Shift* (2016), Brown fuses creative writing with technical writing, rhetoric, and aesthetic to describe a day in the life of a nurse. Brown exemplifies technical writing by simplifying complicated concepts for a non-expert audience even while she is telling a story. Furthermore, *The Shift* discusses issues as various as workplace ethics, informed consent, resource allocation, assessing and addressing suffering, burnout, empathy, workplace communication, technical writing, and others. It also provides an excellent transition in the course from the emphasis on rhetorical aesthetics to the emphasis on (aesthetic) rhetoric. Class discussions invite students to consider what they can learn from Brown about nursing, empathy, health communication, or narrative medicine. This exercise, including the listening practice, helps students prepare and write their reflective assignment on humanities and health.

Students who work together to discover a relationship between the humanities, writing, and health – and to articulate why this relationship matters – develop trust among one another, a trust that is crucial to writing and reading a personal narrative. Because class members need time to develop trust before they write and such a personal narrative – especially a pathography – I believe that a personal narrative assignment is less effective if it is assigned at the beginning of the course. Once students have discovered a relationship between health, the humanities, and writing, and once they trust one another, they are ready to write a personal narrative and share it with the rest of the class.

The personal narrative that students write is a pathography. To introduce pathographies, we discuss Susan Sontag's (1978) statement that illness is "the night-side of life," that "everyone who is born holds dual citizenship, in the kingdom of the well and in the kingdom of the sick," and that while "we all prefer to use only the good passport, sooner or later each of us is obliged, at least for a spell, to identify ourselves as citizens of that other place" (p. 3). I invite students to ponder what it means and what it feels like to be a citizen of "that other place" and when in their lives they have felt like that citizen. They then discuss their experiences in small groups and perform interview exercises as they prepare to write a pathography about an illness that they experienced or that someone close to them experienced. Students choose something that they are comfortable sharing with others.

Pathography combines elements of both biography and *pathos*, the things that people experience and suffer. Writing a pathography can provide students with increased empathy and self-understanding (Hwang et al., 2013). Pathographies also provide a window into people's experiences with illness (Hawkins, 1999), sharing and teaching what it is like to feel, experience, suffer from, and struggle with an illness. Frank's (2013) description of the wounded storyteller's restitution, chaos, and quest narratives that formulate the self can also help students to make sense of how they have oriented their own pathographies. As such, students are invited to be specific about their thoughts, emotions, and responses to the illness; to use their best skills as a storyteller to help others understand and feel what their experiences have taught them; to tell why this experience has helped them decide what they want to do and to be; and to share why it might have influenced and informed their life and goals. These creative, often difficult acts of expression press out – they ex-press (Dewey, 1934) – students' felt experiences into symbols that others can understand and learn from. Writing a personal narrative is also a rhetorical aesthetic act that provides opportunities for self-discovery.

Rhetorical Aesthetics, Listening, and Others

A pedagogy informed by rhetorical aesthetics emphasizes the importance of individuals not only through listening and understanding the experiences of the self but also through listening and understanding the experiences of others. In this section, I describe the following activities that help students listen to and understand the experiences of others: listening to class members read their pathographies, taking a midterm that includes a focus on class members, and performing a simple but memorable listening exercise on a final exam.

The practice of writing and sharing personal compositions is of course passed down from ancient rhetoric pedagogy (see Walker, 2011). To prepare, students who will deliver their pathographies on a given day submit their narratives to a discussion board on a course learning application to which all students have in-class access. Each student reads their pathography while the rest of the class follows along, listening. After the student finishes reading, the other class members take two or three minutes to write a note to the student, thanking them and making other comments. These responses, reactions, and experiences to the narrative are posted to the discussion board, and then the next student reads their narrative. This process of listening to each student read their narrative aloud takes a little more than a week of class periods, but it is worth the time it takes, not just for the learning experiences it provides but also because it emphasizes the importance of listening to and understanding individuals.

Just as *telling* stories promotes self-discovery and learning, so too does *listening* to stories (Coles, 1989). Writing a personal narrative and listening to the personal narratives of other class members can create a community in which students learn to empathize with, trust, and learn from those who make themselves vulnerable. As students prepare to read their personal narratives out loud, word for word, to the rest of the class, they find themselves focusing on saying exactly what they want to say exactly as they want to say it. This focus can improve their writing because they are thinking about their audience and how the audience will receive each and every word, sentence, and paragraph.

A second crucial aspect of this assignment is that the instructor is not exempt from writing and reading aloud a personal narrative several days before other class members begin to read theirs. Through the process of submitting to the assignment, becoming vulnerable, and honestly sharing a personal narrative, the instructor provides a model of what the assignment should look like and sets the stage for other class members As long as the instructor's narrative is honest, sincere, and clear – without overindulging, without calling undue attention to themself, and without using this as an opportunity to show off – the instructor's model can build trust and foster an environment in which other students can become vulnerable as they write about difficult situations they, or their loved ones, have experienced.

Writing a personal narrative, particularly a pathography, and sharing it with other class members can help participants to become poet-professionals who can identify and empathize with others (see Slater, forthcoming, 2023). Some of what class members learn during these exercises is ineffable but nonetheless can be felt. In addition, what students learn is manifested in motivations to inspire, to lift, to edify, to help, to serve, to listen, to understand, and to empathize. Pedagogy based on a rhetorical aesthetic aids this process because participants begin to realize, as Arthur Frank (2013) has written, that "sooner or later, everyone is a wounded storyteller" (p. xxi). By reading personal narratives together as a class, and by honestly and sincerely sharing our stories with one another, we begin to see that our "interests are joined" (Burke, 1969, p. 20). We identify when we see that we are part of the same community. While our experiences differ, our collective attempts to understand one another gives us common ground that helps us to empathize. Our care for and value of people deepens.

Exams That Reinforce the Emphasis on People, Individuals, Listening, and Experience

In a writing course emphasizing health literacies, the most important elements of the class are not concepts – they are people. This hierarchy of importance does not diminish the importance of the subject matter but rather places it in its proper context. Seeing people at the top of a hierarchy of importance can encourage students to *want* to study, learn, and live in accordance with principles that invite all of us to treat people like people and to humanize our care for one another. Emphasizing the story in the first half of the course highlights the idea that some learning experiences – especially those gained from rhetorical aesthetics – are difficult, if not impossible, to measure fully, to test fully, or to report fully. Methods for testing or examining can also provide important teaching experiences – experiences aesthetic and rhetorical that can potentially transform the identity of those who are addressed.

While giving exams in a writing class may seem unusual, especially since papers and projects are weighted heavier than exams, some universities require all courses to have exams. In addition, by making exams into teaching and learning experiences rather than merely testing experiences, instructors can provide students with additional opportunities to transform their identities through a rhetorical aesthetic and prepare them to care for, listen to, and help others. In what follows, I describe only a few sections of the exams that are relevant for building and using a rhetorical aesthetic as part of an underlying pedagogy.

A Midterm That Emphasizes People and Individuals

The class midterm includes three sections, the first of which is simply called "Our Names." This section includes the same number of questions as there are class members. The introduction to this section of the exam asks students to write down the names of all members of the class. Since the humanities are particularly concerned with people, testing students on the names of class members demonstrates the importance of learning and remembering peoples' names. Knowing people's names and using them in respectful ways is the first step in treating people like people – in listening to them, caring for them, and helping them. Students know ahead of time that they will be asked to name each student, so part of studying for the midterm means finding out and remembering class members' names. A class before the midterm can end 5 or 10 minutes early so that students have time to talk to each other and study for the midterm. And since students have been working with each other all along in small groups and with partners, they already know almost everyone. Because seeing a person's face prompts a memory of that person's name, students sit in a circle as they take the midterm, so that they can see everyone else. All they have to do is write down the names of everyone else in the class.

Learning and remembering other class members' names also helps to counteract the tendency towards dehumanization that can sometimes occur in healthcare and other settings. Even in social situations, it has become commonplace to treat people's names lightly, often with the excuse, "I'm terrible with names." But whether or not this problem may stem from something bigger, having a test that has everyone's names on it emphasizes that our names are important, and, by extension, so are we as individuals important. Because students know that they will be tested on one another's names, the idea that people are most important is reinforced. The most important thing in class is not something in the textbook or on a slide. The most important thing in the class is the students. Not only does this activity reinforce this idea, but it also helps to instill in students the notion that everyone is precious, that each person has an intrinsic worth that cannot be measured – and this is one of the most important things that anyone can learn.

A Final Exam That Emphasizes Listening, Understanding, and Experience Over Knowledge

After students write in other, more technical genres like a proposal, SOAP notes, and a formal literature review (with "literature" shifting its meaning from what it meant in the first part of the course), I reinforce the emphasis on individuals and their stories in the final question of the final exam. The last section of the final exam reinforces the idea that knowledge of things and concepts is not more important than but is a means to helping people. The final exam was not weighted as much as the technical research papers, and the last section was not weighted as much as the previous sections. Nevertheless, having such a last section – especially placing it last – reinforced the notion of rhetorical aesthetics that we discussed throughout the course. After several questions that tested student knowledge and application of important course concepts, the last section emphasizes the importance of listening, even when one knows the right answer. Called, "Surprise—Read a Story," the last section provides these instructions:

> Narrative medicine and health humanities comprise an important part of this course and, hopefully, of your own professional development. Given the idea that stories teach us in different but complementary ways, please simply relax and read the following story. After you read the story, answer the final question. That question asks you simply if you have read the story, and the correct answer to the last question is "Yes."

> So, there you go. You know the final answer to the final question. Now all you need to do is read the story and answer. And as you read, think about what this story, and what other stories, can teach you—think about things that *can't* be tested on a final exam …

The ellipsis in the above quotation is included in the instructions as a way of inviting students to ponder what they have learned about the relationship between knowledge, experience, and persuasion – and rhetorical aesthetics. On the next page of the exam, students are presented with a two-and-a-half-page story in which a fictional character suffers but through a changed identity learns to transcend the suffering. After the story, the final question, "Did you read the entire story?" presents students with two options:

A.   Yes
B.   No

I am not interested in whether students get the answer "correct" – after all, students are given the answer in the instructions. More importantly, this question emphasizes listening, trusting, and experience above everything else. The real point of the question, and even the final exam, is *not* about knowledge that is separated from experience. Knowledge is essential, but it cannot supplant genuine listening. Listening is essential, even when we already know the answers. And listening does something, not just for others, but for us: it influences and even changes everyone involved – both the listener and the person being listened to. Listening can potentially transform us as we transcend our differences with another person through an implicit rhetorical aesthetic that lies in the sharing of their story. While knowledge in health literacies is important and absolutely essential, knowledge cannot supplant genuine listening because in order for knowledge to be *valued*, it has to be trusted and even loved. And because genuine listening helps to instill trust, it can help prepare for rhetorical aesthetic identification discussed earlier.

The short story that students read might also be termed a pathography. It may also remind students of the scene at the end of *Wit* (1999) when E. M. Ashford reads to Vivian Bearing the short children's story, Brown's *The runaway bunny* (1942). Stories like these – even children's stories and fairy tales – can provide readers with fantasy, recovery, escape, and consolation and include a joyful eucatastrophe that offers readers hope (see Tolkien, 1983) – a hope that can inspire students as they leave the classroom and turn to other final exams and projects. Above all, the final section of the final exam may seem so strange and even radical that students will, I hope, remember it. They can take this with them wherever they go. It is a gift – a gift of confidence that provides students with an inner strength that I hope will last as they continue to learn to listen to stories and ponder the idea that some learning – perhaps the most important learning – is unquantifiable, ineffable, and unexaminable. (Perhaps not surprisingly, I have yet to see a student's exam that gets this question wrong.)

By emphasizing story above concept, this activity reinforces the idea that each individual, each person involved in health literacies, has a story, and that story matters. Before we try to solve people's problems, we have to genuinely listen to their stories so that we know who they are and how we can help, persuade, teach, and influence them.

Conclusion

Rhetorical-aesthetically-grounded teaching tactics like those I have discussed in this chapter invite students to understand that the real importance lies not in books or reports or instructions or texts, not in papers or documents or multimodal projects, not in concepts or heaps of terms – not even in assignment grades, in grade point averages, or in graduation – but in people: in our fellow human beings who sojourn on earth with us, whether we see them once and never see them again; whether we connect with them on a deeper, more personal and experiential level; or somewhere in between.

The quality of our lives depends on the quality of our own rhetoric and on how we respond to the rhetoric of others (see Booth, 2004). Implicit in all rhetoric is aesthetic, just as implicit in all aesthetic is rhetoric. Rhetorical aesthetic potentially changes who we are – transforms our identities – as we choose to either accept or reject it (or parts of it). As our students not only transform their own identities but also prepare to help others in healthcare settings manage the formation and transformation of their own identities, they need to know how to improve the quality of their rhetoric as they listen to and respond to the rhetoric of others.

Meanwhile, rhetorical aesthetics can provide teachers of health literacies with creative ways of implementing activities and assignments that invite students to act and not be acted upon, encouraging them to treat themselves and others like people and not like objects, circumventing tendencies toward dehumanization, valorizing empathy and genuine listening, and providing people with shared experiences.

Suggestions for Teaching

Health literacies that emphasize increasing the ability of people to find, understand, and use information and services related to health, both for themselves and for others, moves in the right direction. Looking closely at the clause "for themselves and for others" leads to the crucial rhetorical aesthetic and even creative side of health literacies. A rhetorical aesthetic that includes narrative medicine and health humanities provides a groundwork for more technical genres because the rhetorical aesthetic concept of identification helps to emphasize people through listening to the self and listening to others. Exercises that can help students listen include writing in a journal, discovering concepts for themselves, studying literature, and writing a personal narrative. Exercises that can help students listen to others include listening to others, reading the work of others, writing about what others have written, being tested on the names of others, and understanding that people are more important than things. These exercises that emphasize individuals prepare students to focus on their audience when they write and communicate, a key factor in rhetoric and in effective technical communication. My hope is to help all of us to move beyond task-oriented, mechanical, and functional approaches to health literacies and communication.

Many instructors already incorporate a theory of rhetorical aesthetics in their pedagogical methods, but may not do so using the name "rhetorical aesthetics." The following bullet points provide instructors with suggestions for activities that can help students to emphasize people.

- Include excerpts from texts about rhetorical aesthetics. Some of these excerpts, like those from the quintessential rhetorical aesthetic theorist Kenneth Burke, can be found in the references to this chapter. A good place to begin is *A rhetoric of motives* (1969) or "Literature as equipment for living" (1973), in which Burke discusses the aesthetic as a type of symbolic medicine.
- Have students write about their individual experiences.
- Invite students to keep a handwritten journal.
- Include names of individual class members on quizzes or exams.
- Include a unit on narrative medicine that invites students to read and listen to literary texts and perform narrative humility.

References

Anderson, L. W., Krathwol, D. R., Airasian, P. W., Cruikshank, K. A., Mayer, R. E., Pintrich, P. R., Raths, J., & Wittrock, M. C. (2001). *A taxonomy of learning, teaching, and assessing: A revision of Bloom's taxonomy of educational objectives*. Longman.

Berlin, J. A. (1982). Contemporary composition: The major pedagogical theories. *College English*, 44(8), 765–777.

Booth, W. C. (1981). The common aims that divide us; or, is there a "Profession 1981"? *Profession 81*, 13–17.

Booth, W. C. (2004). *The rhetoric of rhetoric: The quest for effective communication*. Blackwell.

Brown, M. W. (1942). *The runaway bunny*. HarperCollins.

Brown, T. (2010). *Critical care: A new nurse faces death, life, and everything in between*. HarperCollins.

Brown, T. (2016). *The shift: One nurse, twelve hours, four patients' lives*. Algonquin.

Burke, K. (1969). *A rhetoric of motives*. University of California Press. (Original work published 1950)

Burke, K. (1966). *Language as symbolic action: Essays on life, literature, and method*. University of California Press.

Burke, K. (1973). Literature as equipment for living. In K. Burke (Ed.), *The philosophy of literary form: Studies in symbolic action* (3rd ed., pp. 49–61). University of California Press.

Burke, K. (1967). Rhetoric—Old and new. In M. Steinmann (Ed.), *New rhetorics* (pp. 59–76). Scribner.

Burke, K. (1931/1968). *Counter-statement*. (3rd ed.). University of California Press.

Burke, K. (1937/1984). *Attitudes toward history*. (3rd ed.). University of California Press.

Campbell, L. (2018). The rhetoric of health and medicine as a "teaching subject": Lessons from the medical humanities and simulation pedagogy. *Technical Communication Quarterly*, 27(1), 7–20.

Charon, R. (2006). *Narrative medicine: Honoring the stories of illness*. Oxford University Press.

Charon, R., Rivera Colón, E., DasGupta, S., Hermann, N., Irvine, C., Marcus, E. R., Spencer, D., & Spiegel, M. (2015). *The principles and practice of narrative medicine*. Oxford University Press.

Cicero, M. T. (2001). *On the ideal orator* (J. M. May & J. Wisse, Trans.). Oxford University Press. (Original work published 55 BCE)

Clark, G. (2015). *Civic jazz: American music and Kenneth Burke on the art of getting along*. University of Chicago Press.

Clark, G. (2004). *Rhetorical landscapes in America: Variations on a theme from Kenneth Burke.* University of South Carolina Press.

Clark, G. (2000). Wayne C. Booth. In M. G. Moran & M. Ballif (Eds.), *Twentieth-century rhetorics and rhetoricians: Critical studies and sources* (pp. 49–61). Greenwood.

Cole, T. R., Carlin, N. S., & Carson, R. A. (2015). *Medical humanities: An introduction.* Cambridge University Press.

Coles, R. (1989). *The call of stories: Teaching and the moral imagination.* Houghton Mifflin.

DasGupta, S. (2008, March). Narrative humility. *Lancet, 371*(9617), 980–981.

Dewey, J. (1934). *Art as experience.* Penguin.

Edson, M. (1999). *Wit.* Farrar, Straus and Giroux.

Ewald, C. (1991). The story of the fairy-tale. In J. Zipes (Ed.), *Spells of enchantment: The wonderous fairy tales of Western culture* (pp. 564–565). Penguin. (Original work published 1909)

Frank, A. W. (2013). *The wounded storyteller: Body, illness, and ethics* (2nd ed.). University of Chicago Press.

Graff, R., & Leff, M. (2005). Revisionist historiography and rhetorical tradition(s). In R. Graff, A. E. Walzer, & J. M. Atwill (Eds.), *The viability of the rhetorical tradition.* State University of New York Press.

Hawkins, A. H. (1999). Pathography: Patient narratives of illness. *Western Journal of Medicine, 171*(2), 127–129.

Heath, M. (2017). Rhetoric and pedagogy. In M. J. MacDonald (Ed.), *The Oxford handbook of rhetorical studies* (pp. 73–83). Oxford University Press.

Hwang, K., Fan, H., & Hwang S. W. (2013). Writing about an experience of illness in medical students. *Advances in Medical Education and Practice, 4*, 151–155.

Mangino, H. (2014). Narrative medicine's role in graduate nursing curricula: Finding and sharing wisdom through story. *Creative Nursing, 20*(3), 191–193.

Paley, K. S. (2001). *I-writing: The politics and practice of teaching first-person writing.* Southern Illinois University Press.

Plato. (2009). Gorgias. In J. Sachs (Trans.), *Gorgias and Rhetoric* (pp. 29–120.). Focus. (Original work published ca. 387 BCE)

Quintilian, M. F. (2001). *The orator's education* (D. A. Russell, Trans.). Harvard University Press. (Original work published ca. 95 CE)

Sheilds, L. E. (2016). Narrative knowing: A learning strategy for understanding the role of stories in nursing practice. *Journal of Nursing Education, 55*(12), 711–714.

Slater, J. (2018). Attitudes of collaborative expectancy: Antithesis, gradatio, and *A rhetoric of motives*, page 58. *Rhetoric Review, 37*(3), 247–258.

Slater, J. (Forthcoming 2023). Pathographies as medicine: Forming empathetic poet-professionals in the health writing classroom. In A. George & L. Weiser (Eds.), *Burke in the classroom.* Parlor Press.

Sontag, S. (1978). *Illness as metaphor.* Farrar, Straus and Giroux.

Tolkien, J. R. R. (1983). On fairy-stories. In C. Tolkien (Ed.), *The monsters and the critics and other essays* (pp. 109–161). HarperCollins.

Walker, J. (2000). *Rhetoric and poetics in antiquity.* Oxford University Press.

Walker, J. (2011). *The genuine teachers of this art: Rhetorical education in antiquity.* University of South Carolina Press.

Westover, T. (2018). *Educated: A memoir.* Random House.

5

CROSS-DISCIPLINARY VACCINE EDUCATION THROUGH A CAMPUS-COMMUNITY PARTNERSHIP

Michael J. Klein

During the fall of 2019, I taught an upper-division undergraduate course called Writing in the Health Sciences. The course is designed for students in a writing-focused discipline to experience firsthand how to effectively communicate on subject matter related to health and wellness, in turn improving their own health literacies and the literacies of those they communicate with. Thus, this course helps students and the clients they serve meet a central focus of the DHHS Healthy People 2030 initiative, which sets "measurable objectives to improve the health and well-being of people nationwide" (U.S. Department of Health and Human Services, n.d.).

The course draws students from our writing, rhetoric, and technical communication (WRTC) major and the cross-disciplinary minors in medical humanities and substance abuse education. This latest iteration also provided symposium credit for students enrolled in the honors college, which increased the number of disciplines the students were drawn from (e.g., biology, chemistry, and media arts).

The course functions as a community-engaged learning course, which is a requirement for the WRTC major. In this type of course, students work with a community partner, which may include a non-academic unit on campus, such as the university health center; a local government agency; or a non-profit. Working in small groups, the students serve as consultants for these community clients, collaborating with them to develop deliverables (e.g., brochures, websites, videos, etc.) that support the mission of the client organization. To do this, students utilized a framework of invention questions based upon the work of Bowden and Scott (Bowdon & Scott, 2002).

Invention serves as the beginning of the writing process: questions developed during this stage help writers better assess their audience and the context of their

DOI: 10.4324/9781003316770-7

communication. In this way, they began the project by assessing the rhetorical situation as a means of understanding the needs of both their client organization and the communities served by that organization. In previous iterations of the course, students have prepared and administered surveys on college student awareness of advanced care directives; redesigned health manuals for participants in a community senior women wellness program; and developed new informational materials for the university health center international travel clinic. While all these projects have been related to health/wellness/medicine, they have not been on the same health topic. For this offering, however, all students worked on a public health writing project, which included strategies for writing across the curriculum (Clark & Fischbach, 2008; Mackenzie, 2018).

Specifically, the students addressed issues related to vaccines in Virginia. Partnering with two local agencies—Healthy Families and the Central Shenandoah Health District—students investigated aspects of the ongoing debate about the safety and efficacy of vaccines, developing strategies and methods for providing information to the local community. Specifically, this pedagogical approach implemented several specific changes:

- Including students from various majors in an upper-division health writing course
- Partnering with faculty and clinicians from health-related fields in teaching the course
- Engaging with community partners and focusing on discrete aspects of a specific health-related crisis
- Providing students the opportunity to create materials that could have a positive impact on stakeholders in the crisis, including clinicians, patients, policy makers, etc.

By utilizing these changes, I demonstrate in this specific case how a rhetorically grounded, cross-disciplinary approach to health communication can assist agencies in informing their constituents about vaccines by increasing their public health literacies.

The Pre-COVID Vaccine Debate

(NOTE: Because this course took place before the COVID-19 pandemic, discussions of COVID vaccines and the resistance to taking them did not come up in the class and are beyond the scope of this narrative. However, many of the issues the students addressed are as relevant, or even more so, as they relate to people's resistance to taking the COVID vaccines.)

The first anti-vaccine movement was aimed at the first vaccine: the smallpox vaccine developed by Edward Jenner in the early 19th century (Ryan, 2019). Thus, vaccines and people's resistance/hesitancy to taking them have gone hand-in-hand for over two hundred years. The current debate about the efficacy and safety of vaccines, especially for infants and children, while just one in a string of historical debates dating back to Jenner's first vaccine, began with the 1998 Wakefield et al article in *The Lancet* (Wakefield et al., 1998). Wakefield and his team described "intestinal abnormalities" in all 12 children vaccinated with the MMR (measles, mumps, and rubella) vaccine, as well as postulating a link with autism for those vaccinated. The article was later retracted by *The Lancet* in 2010, as the UK's General Medical Council found that Wakefield acted unethically (Triggle, 2010).

But even with the research withdrawn, and several subsequent studies finding no connection between the vaccines and autism, anti-vaxxers (as they are labeled by those who are proponents of vaccines) still urge parents to investigate the linkage before vaccinating their children. In fact, over the past two decades, the debate has shifted from pro-/anti-vaccine to responsibility of the public/ individual choice. Many of those labeled as anti-vaxxers reject the designation, instead preferring the term vaccine "hesitancy" (Larson et al., 2014). Additionally, many state that they are pro-vaccine (and, thus, not anti-science), but are reticent to allow the government to take away decision-making related to vaccinations from individual parents and guardians (Smith, 2019). Even though a large majority of scientists, medical clinicians, and research publications point to these vaccines as being both safe and effective, many vaccine-hesitant individuals still would rather face the increased risk of infection rather than the much less-likely risk of vaccine serious side effects, an action that could have devastating effects worldwide in the years to come (World Health Organization, 2019).

Such a move to reject vaccines that have a long track record of affording protection from disease can have a debilitating effect on populations. This can subsequently be compounded by public health departments not being attuned to the needs, values, and norms of their constituents. For example, the members of the Somali community in the Twin Cities region of Minnesota traditionally had high vaccine rates. However, as the anti-vaccine movement gained strength in the early 2000s, this community was adversely affected by listening to, and in some cases adhering to, their pronouncements about the dangers of vaccines. After vaccination rates dropped dramatically, a large-scale outbreak of measles occurred, a disease usually held in check by the MMR vaccine. This confusion on the part of the Somali community members was compounded by the lack of cultural awareness on the part of the local health department, especially by ad-dressing the community only in English and inadequately addressing the causes of the vaccine hesitancy (Aziz et al., 2018).

Such incidents can be remedied by having technical communicators play a larger role in disseminating information in public health campaigns. In fact, practitioners in the fields of technical communication and the rhetoric of health and medicine have examined the public debate over vaccines in recent years, using various methodological approaches, including rhetorical analysis of college student responses to a vaccine survey, and interviews with physicians about their perspectives on vaccines and disease (Hausman, 2017; Lawrence, 2014; Lawrence, 2018). My chapter extends the analysis of the way vaccines and vaccinations are framed by clinicians by following the work of under-graduates in producing educational materials, under the auspices of local healthcare agencies, for individuals who might be hesitant about vaccinating their children or receiving vaccines themselves. Vaccine literacies, then, are an important component of health literacies.

The Course and Clients

Writing in the Health Sciences is an upper-division, undergraduate course ori-ginally designed for WRTC at James Madison University. It is designated a community-based learning course for our curriculum, one of four such courses with this designation. WRTC majors are required to select one of the four courses to complete their degree. Because of the nature of professional and technical communication, the curriculum committee revising our degree struc-ture ten years ago recognized the need for students to have formal training with clients before they began their capstone internship. In my class, for example, students work in teams of approximately five students, each spending an average of five hours per week for ten weeks working on client projects. This work is supplemented by readings and class discussions on topics relevant to professional writing, healthcare communication, and project management.

Additionally, every few weeks I hold a project debrief with the students. At this time, students can openly discuss issues they're having with the projects, the clients, or other aspects of the process. While the students appreciate the op-portunity to hold these "bitch sessions" as a means of letting off steam, I use them as a way to discuss issues that will often arise when working for clients, either internal or external to one's organization. For example, clients may not always listen to suggestions made by them, even if these suggestions are based upon sound rhetorical or design theory, instead choosing another option. These teaching moments help students understand that what they are going through is not unique; rather, they can expect to experience similar situations in their professional careers. By learning that their peers often have the same problems and being reassured that such problems are more commonplace than one would expect, students grow closer to their group members and group cohesion often increases. The students begin to see themselves as professional communicators, realizing that being a student does not preclude one from being a working professional.

During the fall, members of the class worked with two local agencies. The first was Healthy Families of Shenandoah and Page Counties, which this author had a long-term relationship with due to previous pedagogical collaborations. Healthy Families "empowers families by connecting them to community resources and offering in-home services" and is a program of the Institute for Innovation in Health and Human Services (IIHHS) at JMU (Shenandoah & Page County Healthy Families, n.d.).

Healthy Families has been active in its community for 20 years, serving over 500 families during that time. These two rural counties are comprised of predominantly White, working-class families with a high school education; approximately 10% of the residents do not have healthcare (U.S. Census Bureau, 2021a; U.S. Census Bureau, 2021b).

Healthy Families asked for a team of students to work on vaccine education. Previously, Healthy Families has "tried to educate parents as to the importance of vaccinations while trying to dispel fears of Autism and other terrible side effects. The focus now needs to be more on what happens if children AREN'T immunized" (Y.H. Frazier, email communication, August 5, 2019). To accomplish this, Healthy Families asked a group of students to do the following:

- Do some research (particularly state/local) regarding measles, mumps, rubella (MMR vaccine), Diphtheria, Tetanus, Pertussis (DTaP), Polio (IPV), Chickenpox (Varicella), Hepatitis A and B cases in the last 3-5 years, as well as symptoms/deaths from these.
- Find out if local doctors are turning away children who aren't vaccinated.
- Find out how local child care, preschools, and public schools handle children who haven't had state 'required' vaccines, including concerns for staff safety (what if a staff person is pregnant or has a compromised immune system?)
- Create talking points/script home visitors (and others) can use in talking with parents to help them decide if they are prepared for the roadblocks not immunizing can bring, and how they will protect their children if they are unimmunized- looking long term. It can be difficult to "catch up," I believe, if parents decide at age 5 to begin getting immunizations. (Y.H. Frazier, email communication, August 5, 2019).

The other students worked with the Central Shenandoah Health District (CSHD), one of the 35 health districts that comprise the Virginia Department of Health. This client was identified as having a health communication need through JMU's Community Service-Learning Office. The mission of CSHD is to "[p]rotect and promote the health and well-being of residents in the Central Shenandoah Valley" (Virginia Department of Health, 2022a). CSHD is "comprised of seven health departments that serve the counties of Augusta, Bath, Highland, Rockbridge and Rockingham … [and] provide[s] numerous services to approximately 293,000 citizens" (Virginia Department of Health, 2022b).

CSHD asked for a team of students to design materials related to the myths and facts of the influenza (flu) vaccine. CSHD sees the flu as a "substantial burden on the health and wellbeing of the citizens of Virginia," due to the "2,222 cases of pneumonia and influenza related deaths in the Commonwealth of Virginia during the 2018-19 flu season" (L.L. Wight, email communication, August 19, 2019). Specifically, CSHD wanted students to "create a digital PSA about common myths and facts about the influenza vaccine to provide community members with scientific information about the vaccine so community members can make an informed decision when deciding whether or not to get the vaccine" (L.L. Wight, email communication, August 19, 2019).

Based upon these requests, the members of the class indicated their choice to me of which client they wished to work. While I tried to honor their choices, I did take several things into consideration when forming the teams. First, I wanted there to be a mix of majors, with each team having a least one WRTC major, one science (biology or psychology) major, and one health-related (health sciences or kinesiology) major. Second, I made sure that the teams had both honors and non-honors students. Third, I ensured that team members were a mix of sophomores, juniors, and seniors, reflecting different levels of training and expertise.

By using these criteria, team members would be working with students from different disciplines. This would accomplish a number of things. First, students have to rely on their team members' expertise to complete in-class assignments and to produce client deliverables. Students would need to rely on one another to be successful because the projects required expertise in conducting scientific research, a knowledge of the effects of immunization in populations and individuals and utilizing rhetorical strategies for communicating with general audiences. This would provide them with a better understanding of working in teams, something they will do extensively in their careers. Second, and more importantly, students would take ownership of their area of expertise, functioning as a subject matter expert for their specific area in completing the client's work. This would provide them with the experience of professionalization by developing their ethos with colleagues.

Course Assignments

Students completed a number of assignments that would support their work with the clients within a service-learning environment. First, as in Jarron Slater's course (see Chapter 4), students kept a weekly reflection journal to record their thoughts and experiences. Reflection is an essential component to the service-learning course, allowing both students and instructor to better asses the learning taking place (Eyler, 2002; Molee et al., 2010). The students also composed a reflection essay for their final assignment, in which they reflected upon the similarities and differences between a traditional writing class and one that partners with community clients.

Second, students composed a task analysis of their client and projects (see box 5.1). The task analysis, adapted from Bowdon and Scott's discussion of the rhetorical situation (Bowdon & Scott, 2002), allowed students to situate their project within four larger elements: writer, audience, text and subject, and contextual spheres of production, distribution, and reception. Working with their clients, students produced a short (300-400 word) analysis for each of the four elements by drawing upon standard invention questions (e.g., what are your roles as author? and who is your primary target audience?). This task analysis further served as means of making appropriate rhetorical choices when producing the actual deliverables for their clients.

BOX 5.1   TASK ANALYSIS PROMPT

Working in your client groups, you will perform a task analysis using the invention questions found in the Bowden and Scott chapter we read for class (reproduced on the second page of this prompt). Do not simply respond to each question individually. Rather, use the questions in each section, which are organized into core elements of the rhetorical situation, to help you produce a coherent analysis (of 300–400 words) for **each** element. If you are working to produce more than one text, choose the primary text you will be revising/producing to respond to the relevant questions.

Third, students produced a portfolio that included agreed-upon deliverables for their clients. The portfolio, which comprised the largest part of their work for the course, also included a letter of transmittal to the client summarizing their deliverables, as well as a presentation about the entire project process made at the end of the course to their client.

While the clients had a type of deliverable in mind at the beginning for the project, students fleshed out these initial conceptions in producing the final work. First, they drew upon the associated task analysis. They also used an iterative process in working with the clients, sharing drafts with the client, and making changes based upon feedback throughout the semester. Finally, students presented their work to other members of the class, soliciting comments regarding appropriateness for the intended audience.

Client Deliverables

In this section, I briefly describe and analyze the rhetorical choices made by the students in producing their primary deliverables.

Healthy Families

The students working with Healthy Families produced a Vaccine FAQ Sheet for the use of Healthy Family staff in home visits. This document can be used by home visitors (and others) in talking with parents to help them decide if they are prepared for the roadblocks not immunizing can bring and how they will protect their children if they are unimmunized. It also included references to the sources where it drew its information.

In order to make the information accessible for its audience, the students utilized common, informal language in an FAQ format. When informal language was not appropriate, they used language appropriate for their respective audiences. This is especially true for the information provided about the types of diseases targeted by vaccines. For example, when discussing the side effects of polio, the document explains that paralysis is when "you can't move your arm or leg." The use of language in this way has a secondary benefit of making it easier for the Healthy Families staff members to explain the concepts orally to clients while reading a script.

Coupled with the type of language was an FAQ model for the document. Drawing upon information gathered from years of experience Healthy Families had in working with their clients, the students drafted the types of questions usually asked by clients and then coupled these with typical responses. This type of format couples nicely with the writing style the students used. For example, the first question is "What are the consequences of not getting your child vaccinated?"; one of the responses is "Your kids might not be able to attend public school …." This use of second-person language, in which the author addresses the listener/reader directly, makes the information clearer and more relevant, and it is commonly found in technical communication. The question-and-answer format uses the term "your," making the message pertinent to the audience. It also uses colloquial language like "kid" in the response, as this is a term many parents use for their children.

In composing the questions and answers, the students followed the Healthy Families directive to inform but not advocate. This distinction is often hard to make; after all, the selection of the information one provides is a rhetorical choice. In speaking with the students during one of our class sessions, they stated that they had decided to only use information from reliable sources: medical practitioners and state agencies. They would also present information without using a call-to-action. That is, they would lay out the facts and let the audience come to their own conclusion. For example, in crafting a response to the question "Why should I get this vaccine," the students drew upon a real-life example of a four-year-old, Amanda Kanowitz, who died of influenza (The Amanda Kanowitz Foundation, n.d.).

The implicit message is that your child could end up like Amanda; however, it is up to the audience to draw this conclusion for themselves. Told as a narrative, the story of Amanda's death provides an example of concrete consequences for not vaccinating for influenza, but in a non-judgmental or paternalistic way.

Central Shenandoah Health District

The students working with CSHD produced a 3-minute digital PSA that would be shown in the lobbies of their offices across the region (Central Shenandoah Health District, 2020). The PSA discusses common myths and facts about the influenza vaccine in order to provide community members with scientific information about the vaccine so they can make an informed decision when deciding whether to get the vaccine. As with the Healthy Families project, the digital PSA presents information without a significant amount of persuasion.

The students took a number of steps to appeal to their audience. First, they used plain language coupled with simple imagery to explain concepts. For example, in explaining the types of vaccines available, they refer to them as "the flu shot" and "the flu nasal spray," displaying a needle-tipped syringe and a nose, respectively.

Second, the students used a call-and-response format, with statements labeled as myths, followed by a question and an answer. For example, a placard appears with the language "Myth 1 It is possible to get the flu from the flu vaccine." The video then provides some context by discussing the two types of vaccines available (see above) followed by a question: "Then why can someone still get sick?" Drawing upon information the video states is from the Centers for Disease Control and Prevention (CDC), it provides three explanations for this: infection due to another virus or a bacterium; infection before the flu vaccine; or the vaccine containing the wrong flu strain. The other two myths are introduced and dispelled in a similar fashion throughout the rest of the video. In this way, the students provided specific information in both narrative and visual form, from a trusted source, and appropriate for their intended audience.

Third, and equally important, the video uses imagery of a wide variety of individuals: men and women, babies, toddlers, teens, adults, and the elderly. The individuals also represent a wide variety of ethnicities. Because the CSHD serves the needs of a range of individuals, the students wanted to make sure that the end user would see themselves in the individuals portrayed in the video. In doing so, they increased the likelihood that the viewers would pay attention and identify with the information provided (Beagley, 2011; Singleton & Krause, 2009).

Outcomes and Takeaways

The client response to the work produced was positive, but not without some suggestions for improvement. Healthy Families commented that "The [initial] meeting with the students was very professional and appropriate," but also stated that she "would have liked at bit more interaction and follow-up" (Y.H. Frazier, email communication, December 16, 2019). Similarly, CSHD stated that while communication was "relatively easy," she was concerned with the choice of the platform the group ultimately used for their video as it was not free (L.L. Wight, email communication, January 6, 2020).

These responses accurately capture the overall impressions I had of how the projects unfolded. In this section, I endeavor to comment on what went well, what needs to be improved in future iterations of the course, and what other instructors can take away from this experience.

Positive Outcomes

Using groups of students with diverse educational and professional experiences proved to be beneficial in many ways. I offer these to readers as a rationale for adopting these types of methods in their own courses.

First, because the students came from different disciplinary backgrounds, they were able to function as knowledge experts in their respective fields, establishing their ethos in the process. This allowed them to serve as peer instructors to the other members of their group; in return, they learned from their peers about other aspects of the project. For example, WRTC students understood the rhetorical process before entering the class. This afforded them the opportunity to help their groupmates learn about this vital constituent of the writing process. Conversely, health science students, because of their initially higher health literacies, knew the most reliable and accurate resources to draw upon for information, making the materials they produced credible and, ultimately, more effective. This reciprocal peer learning provided them with authentic opportunities to work together as a team.

Second, this learning approach provided them with an accurate view of what working in a professional environment is like. Almost no occupation, including writing, is done in isolation. Writers depend on editors, content specialists, and peers in creating materials for their audiences. For example, in working on an educational health video, a writer could collaborate with a healthcare specialist to fact-check research on vaccines; coordinate with a videographer to storyboard scenes; and have an editor review her script before shooting begins. This type of career preparation is an invaluable opportunity for students before they enter the professional workplace, as they learn that working with others is an essential component of becoming effective communicators.

Third, a diverse group of students working on a project leads to diverse perspectives and solutions to issues that arise. Different disciplines not only deal with different subject matter; they also employ distinctive modes of inquiry. For example, students in the humanities learn methodologies for exploring the world that are different from those learned by students in the natural sciences: the humanities (usually) use data derived from qualitative studies while the natural sciences (usually) utilize data gathered from quantitative research. Allowing students to experience these varied perspectives firsthand provides them with a rich tapestry of ideas to draw upon when confronting challenges that inevitably arise in composing complex documents for various audiences.

Needs Improvement

Based on feedback from the clients and my own observations, there are two areas that I need to attend to in future iterations of the course. I offer these to readers as issues to consider in adopting these methods.

First, communication between students and their clients needs improvement. The irony of poor communication being demonstrated in a writing course is not lost on me. However, in a course such as this, there are more communication networks than usual. For example, in a traditional class where students just do their own work individually, communication is between the teacher and the students. When students work in groups, then the communication network expands—students communicate within groups and with the instructor. Finally, when students work in groups with external clients, the types of communication further expand—students communicate within groups, with the instructor, and with their clients.

Communication with the clients introduces issues students have yet to encounter. For example, students are used to instructors responding to inquiries in a timely fashion, usually within one or two days; this might be even more frequently given the number of course meetings conducted each week. However, students may not see clients on a regular schedule. And the student work groups are not the only stakeholders the clients need to concern themselves with. As I pointed out to my students, clients are working full-time and have many projects they need to manage.

Managing all of this communication becomes challenging for students, especially when much of it is done via electronic means. Even though groups had elected one of their members to conduct all the communication with the client—in order to eliminate communication missteps—further steps need to be taken. Thus, in the future, I will be employing additional steps to help eliminate these problems.

Students will develop a detailed project plan in consultation with the client at the beginning of the project. This is more than just receiving a list of deliverables, as the plan will incorporate both the client's needs and assumptions of the work to be undertaken. Additionally, to ensure that the project progresses smoothly, the students will need to hold weekly phone or Zoom sessions with their clients to keep them abreast of their progress and receive feedback on the materials they have submitted. These weekly scheduled meetings hold both the students *and* the clients accountable.

The second issue, while it relates directly to the issue of communication, is more rhetorical than logistical. Novice health professional communicators often focus on creating materials for an audience: the end user. However, they must always be cognizant of the fact they are dealing with multiple audiences: the client and the end user. Navigating the needs of multiple audiences must be something that I am much more explicit about discussing throughout the course.

While the students did consider multiple audiences in creating their task analyses, they failed to continuously refer back to this document after they began the work on the deliverables.

One way to alleviate this issue is to keep the task analysis relevant to them throughout the entire course by having them treat it as a living document. While an initial draft will be turned in and evaluated by me early in the class, I will now require groups to continuously update the document as the semester proceeds. This will keep them engaged with the matters they initially identified as well as provide them with the opportunity to make iterative changes as the projects unfold.

Conclusion

As I write this, we are 2 years into the worst pandemic of the past 100 years. The way we live and learn has dramatically changed, and the way we go about communicating about health (and non-health) issues has taken on a new importance. And the way we teach students has also changed for many of us: face-to-face classes have been replaced by online instruction that includes virtual interaction via online video lectures, Zoom classroom meetings, and discussion boards.

But with all these changes, some things remain the same. The response to COVID vaccines, developed in a year after the initial outbreak in the United States, has met even greater resistance than childhood vaccines did in previous years. Ludicrous claims of tracking chips and monitoring systems being injected along with the vaccine abound, as do claims that the virus causes an infection just like a cold (Capritto, 2020). What is evident from this is that increased health literacy for the general populace is paramount to fighting this disease.

Thus, there are some consistencies to the pedagogical approaches I take as I continue teaching this course. New challenges are sure to crop up, but these can be anticipated or accommodated. What will not change is using a strong rhetorical foundation and diverse student population in the course to meet the needs of clients, improve health literacies in both students and the general populace, and train the next generation of health communication professionals.

References

Aziz, F., & Miles, S. H. (2018). Measles, autism and vaccination in the Minnesota Somali community. *Minnesota Medicine*, January/February, 101(1), 30–33.

Beagley, L. (2011). Educating patients: Understanding barriers, learning styles, and teaching techniques. *Journal of PeriAnesthesia Nursing*, 26(5), 331–337. 10.1016/j.jopan. 2011.06.002

Bowdon, M., & Scott, B. (2002). *Service learning in technical and professional communication (Part of the Allyn & Bacon Series in Technical Communication)* (1st ed.). Longman.

Capritto, A. (2020, December 16). *Microchips and mandatory shots: Don't fall for these coronavirus vaccine myths*. CNET. Retrieved July 12, 2022, from https://www.cnet.com/health/microchips-and-mandatory-shots-dont-fall-for-these-coronavirus-vaccine-myths/

Central Shenandoah Health District. (2020, May 27). *Flu Vaccine Myths and Facts [Video]*. YouTube. https://youtu.be/8zcdwOGsTH4

Clark, I. L., & Fischbach, R. (2008). Writing and Learning in the Health Sciences: Rhetoric, Identity, Genre, and Performance. *The WAC Journal*, 19(1), 15–28. 10.37514/wac-j.2008.19.1.02

Eyler, J. (2002). Reflection: Linking service and learning-linking students and communities. *Journal of Social Issues*, 58(3), 517–534. 10.1111/1540-4560.00274

Hausman, B. L. (2017). Immunity, modernity, and the biopolitics of vaccination resistance. *Configurations*, 25(3), 279–300. 10.1353/con.2017.0020

Healthy People | health.gov. (n.d.). Healthy People. Retrieved July 12, 2022, from https://health.gov/our-work/national-health-initiatives/healthy-people

Larson, H. J., Jarrett, C., Eckersberger, E., Smith, D. M., & Paterson, P. (2014). Understanding vaccine hesitancy around vaccines and vaccination from a global perspective: A systematic review of published literature, 2007–2012. *Vaccine*, 32(19), 2150–2159. 10.1016/j.vaccine.2014.01.081

Lawrence, H. Y. (2014). Healthy bodies, toxic medicines: College students and the rhetorics of flu vaccination. *The Yale Journal of Biology and Medicine*, 87(4), 423–437.

Lawrence, H. Y. (2018). When patients question vaccines: Considering vaccine communication through a material rhetorical approach. *Rhetoric of Health & Medicine*, 1(1–2), 161–178. 10.5744/rhm.2018.1010

Mackenzie, S. L. C. (2018). Writing for public health: Strategies for teaching writing in a school or program of public health. *Public Health Reports*, 133(5), 614–618. 10.1177/0033354918785374

Molee, L. M., Henry, M. E., Sessa, V. I., & McKinney-Prupis, E. R. (2010). Assessing learning in service-learning courses through critical reflection. *Journal of Experiential Education*, 33(3), 239–257. 10.5193/jee33.3.239

Ryan, Y. (2019, April 2). *Vaccination and the media – A 19th century debate*. The Newsroom Blog. Retrieved July 12, 2022, from https://blogs.bl.uk/thenewsroom/2019/04/vaccination-and-the-media-a-19th-century-debate.html

Shenandoah & Page County Healthy Families. (n.d.). *Shenandoah & Page County Healthy Families: About Us*. Healthy Families Shenandoah & Page County. Retrieved July 12, 2022, from https://shenandoahpage.wixsite.com/healthyfamilies/about-us

Singleton, K., & Krause, E. (2009). Understanding cultural and linguistic barriers to health literacy. *OJIN: The Online Journal of Issues in Nursing*, 14(3), 4–9. 10.3912/ojin.vol14no03man04

Smith, T. C. (2019, June 17). *Jessica Biel says she supports vaccines — which is exactly what antivaxxers say*. NBC News. Retrieved July 12, 2022, from https://www.nbcnews.com/think/opinion/jessica-biel-says-she-supports-vaccines-which-exactly-what-anti-ncna1017886

The Amanda Kanowitz Foundation. (n.d.). *The Amanda Kanowitz Foundation*. Retrieved July 12, 2022, from http://www.amandakfoundation.org

Triggle, N. (2010, January 28). *BBC News - MMR scare doctor "acted unethically", panel finds*. BBC. Retrieved July 12, 2022, from http://news.bbc.co.uk/1/hi/health/8483865.stm

U.S. Census Bureau. (2021a). *U.S. Census Bureau QuickFacts: Page County, Virginia.* Census Bureau QuickFacts. Retrieved July 12, 2022, from https://www.census.gov/quickfacts/pagecountyvirginia

U.S. Census Bureau. (2021b). *U.S. Census Bureau QuickFacts: Shenandoah County, Virginia.* Census Bureau QuickFacts. Retrieved July 12, 2022, from https://www.census.gov/quickfacts/shenandoahcountyvirginia

U.S. Department of Health and Human Services. (n.d.). *Healthy People 2030 | health.gov.* Healthy People 2030. Retrieved July 12, 2022, from https://health.gov/healthypeople

Virginia Department of Health. (2022a). *Central Shenandoah Health District.* Retrieved July 12, 2022, from https://www.vdh.virginia.gov/central-shenandoah/

Virginia Department of Health. (2022b). *About Us.* Central Shenandoah Health District. Retrieved July 12, 2022, from https://www.vdh.virginia.gov/central-shenandoah/contact-us/

Wakefield, A., Murch, S., Anthony, A., Linnell, J., Casson, D., Malik, M., Berelowitz, M., Dhillon, A., Thomson, M., Harvey, P., Valentine, A., Davies, S., & Walker-Smith, J. (1998). RETRACTED: Ileal-lymphoid-nodular hyperplasia, non-specific colitis, and pervasive developmental disorder in children. *The Lancet*, 351(9103), 637–641. 10.1016/s0140-6736(97)11096-0

World Health Organization. (2019). *Ten threats to global health in 2019.* Retrieved July 12, 2022, from https://www.who.int/news-room/spotlight/ten-threats-to-global-health-in-2019

PART II
Programs

6

CONTEXT MATTERS: IDENTIFYING STRATEGIC OPPORTUNITIES TO SUPPORT HEALTH LITERACIES THROUGH WRITING INTERVENTIONS

Lucy Bryan Malenke

Since the Writing Across the Curriculum (WAC) movement began popularizing writing as a tool for learning in any discipline in the 1970s and 1980s, undergraduate programs have increasingly used writing to assess learning and to facilitate a variety of literacies involving critical thinking, inquiry, analysis, and self-reflection. An outgrowth of WAC, the Writing in the Disciplines (WID) movement has also inspired programs to teach and assign writing tasks that students are likely to encounter in graduate programs, on the job market, or in their professions (Mackenzie, 2018), including the health professions.

Much as the *National Action Plan to Improve Health Literacy* directs organizations, educators, and healthcare providers to understand their contexts of care (HHS, 2010), it is vital for WAC/WID program administrators to understand the agents, structures, and relationships that shape their contexts of instruction. Program administrators must then apply this information as they develop writing initiatives that can support the development of students' health literacies, which I understand here as both individual and organizational. Asking questions about the state of writing in a program is where Oermann et al. (2015) recommended that faculty begin, and Melzer (2013), a composition scholar and coordinator of a WAC program, has suggested that administrators seeking to evaluate, transform, or institute a writing initiative use Critical Systems Thinking (CST) to better understand their contexts.

CST is a transdisciplinary analytical approach to understanding the characteristics of systems; it facilitates problem-solving within systems through targeted structural changes. Melzer (2013) advocated constructing a map of the educational system and its underlying ideologies in order to locate "points of leverage where even small changes will affect the entire system" (p. 75). He also cautioned that transforming complex systems and the conceptual

DOI: 10.4324/9781003316770-9

models that drive them takes time. Although Melzer's (2013) focus was on campus-wide writing initiatives, CST has the potential to benefit individual programs, departments, or even classes, all of which operate within complex educational structures.

Background for the Present Study

The need to improve the writing skills of students interested in behavioral and health fields drove the creation of my faculty line – a liaison position within the writing center at a regional, public university. This experimental joint appointment was a response to requests for enhanced writing and instructional support for the 5,400 students and 160 faculty in the university's largest college, which prepares students to enter professions including counseling, nursing, occupational therapy, public health, physical therapy, social work, and speech-language pathology.

I stepped into this liaison role in the fall of 2014, knowing that I would need to export writing expertise into the college and import disciplinary expertise into the writing center through some combination of teaching, tutoring, tutor training, presentations, workshops, and faculty development – but it was not apparent which needs were most pressing or what approaches would be effective, feasible, and sustainable. As far as I could tell, students were not required to complete any writing-intensive classes beyond first-year composition, and no curricular initiatives to develop field-specific written communication skills existed within the college or its individual departments. Still, the creation of my position indicated that students were not only writing in the college's nine majors but also struggling, in some capacity, with their writing tasks.

In the first months of the job, I began asking questions about the state of writing in the college: How much and what kinds of writing are students doing? What discipline-specific writing instruction, if any, do students receive in their major classes? What are students' barriers to success as writers in their disciplines? What are faculty members' perceptions of student writing and attitudes toward writing instruction? I realized that I would need to develop a formal mechanism for answering my questions and that the most effective and sustainable approaches to serving the college would be grounded in empirical research, not just anecdotal evidence. In other words, I wanted to mirror the commitment to evidence-based practice that I saw in the students, faculty, and departments I'd been hired to serve.

Thus, I set out to acquire the kind of contextual knowledge Oermann et al. (2015) and Melzer (2013) described. However, I struggled to find models and empirical instruments that I could use to explore my institutional context. As a result, I decided to create a set of research instruments that would help me explore the state of writing in departments and programs in the college. My ultimate goal was to identify needs that might act as "impact opportunities," where tailored interventions were likely to bring about meaningful changes and to last.

In designing these instruments, I drew inspiration from surveys of faculty perceptions, attitudes, and pedagogical practices used early in the WAC/WID movements to prepare for the establishment of university-wide writing programs (Duke, 1982; Maimon & Nodine, 1978), as well as studies of disciplinary genres and contexts from composition and WAC scholars (Epstein, 1999; Weiser, 1999; Zerger, 1997). The findings can be understood as a glimpse into a kind of organizational health literacy in the college, given the students' majors and the faculty's professional backgrounds.

Methods

To explore the state of writing in a particular academic program or department, I created a mixed-methods approach that employed surveys and interviews. The pilot study described below was approved by the Institutional Review Board (Protocol # 15–0373) and took place in the spring of 2015 in the health sciences major at my institution. (In the next chapter, Yuko Taniguchi and colleagues discuss the health science program at the University of Minnesota Rochester, providing additional perspectives.)

Participants

A logical choice for a pilot study was the undergraduate health sciences major, the largest major in the college I serve and one of the largest at the university. At the time, it had more than 1,000 declared majors, many of whom planned to enroll in graduate or professional programs in occupational therapy, physical therapy, physician assistant studies, public health, medicine, and other health professions.

I chose to focus on the perspectives of faculty, not students, in part to manage the scope of the study. Moreover, while students come and go, faculty tend to be more enduring variables in the complex systems in which writing and writing instruction occur. They are more likely to be familiar with the history of a program, its administrative structure, and its values. Additionally, interventions that involve faculty are likely to remain in the system for longer and, ideally, to impact multiple student cohorts as well as the institutional culture.

I sent an email soliciting participation in this pilot study to the 44 faculty members in the Health Sciences Department who, between the summer of 2014 and spring of 2015, taught classes in the health sciences major core curriculum or in one of the major's three concentrations – health studies, health assessment and promotion, and public health education. Ultimately, 22 faculty members agreed to take part in the study. Two of those participants withdrew after beginning the study because they did not use writing in their health sciences major classes, resulting in a final participation rate of 45% ($n = 20$).

The participant pool included full-time and part-time faculty with teaching experience ranging from less than one year to more than 15 years.

Within the specified time frame, they taught 19 different courses in the major at the 100, 200, 300, and 400 levels. All participants used at least one writing assignment in their classes. These assignments included in-class writing activities, online discussion boards, reflection papers, position papers, personal statements, letters to legislators, analytical essays, critical reviews, case studies, annotated bibliographies, literature reviews, empirical research studies, and health promotion program plans.

Surveys

In the first phase of the study, each participant received an online Qualtrics survey (Appendix A). The survey used short answer and multiple-choice questions to collect demographic information, to determine how much and what kinds of writing participants assign in their classes, to investigate their relationship with the writing center, and to ascertain what instruction, resources, and feedback they provide for writing assignments. Early in the survey, participants responded to an open-ended question that asked what qualities they think characterize good writing in their discipline. Following that question, the instrument requested that participants rate their average student's proficiency level in 24 writing and writing-related abilities (e.g., organization, accurate citations, and ability to synthesize information and ideas) on a four-point Likert scale (poor, fair, good, excellent). This portion of the survey had excellent internal consistency (Cronbach's α = .938). Participants were asked to select and rank their top five grading considerations from the same list of abilities. The survey also measured participants' attitudes toward writing instruction, their students' writing, and their own writing by asking them to respond to a series of 17 statements using a five-point Likert scale (strongly agree to strongly disagree). Examples of statements in this series include: "Students should be required to do more writing as part of the health sciences major" and "When grading papers, I feel the need to comment on every error."

Interviews

After completing the survey, each participant met with me for a one-on-one, semi-structured interview in a private location. During interviews, they responded to 10 pre-determined, open-ended questions (Appendix B) about:

- Participants' general perceptions of the state of writing in the major;
- Their impressions of students' writing abilities, preparation, attitudes, and barriers to success;
- The writing assignments they used, as well as their purposes or learning objectives;

- The strategies and resources they used to help students improve as writers;
- What they hoped students would get out of visits to the Writing Center;
- What kinds of support they wanted with regard to writing instruction or their own writing projects.

Data Analysis

I exported the quantitative survey data into SPSS. Additionally, I exported participants' qualitative short-answer responses about what characterizes good writing in their discipline into NVivo9, where I classified them into 17 writing ability categories (Appendix C).

The bulk of the data came from the interviews, which I transcribed and imported into NVivo9.

During transcription, I made a list of common topics and trends observed within the data, such as "expectations and standards for students," "perceived problems in student writing," and "teaching practices and strategies." This list became the basis of the thematic "nodes" used for qualitative analysis of the interviews. During the coding process, I refined and expanded my list of themes and organized them into hierarchies. The themes and sub-themes identified in the interviews, as well as the number of participants and coded references corresponding to each theme, are available in Appendix D. For the purposes of comparison, nodes were also assigned to each participant, each interview question, each course, and each assignment type. In order to ensure consistency and accuracy in coding, I reviewed each interview a minimum of three times and verified the selections coded at each node. I then considered the trends revealed by the survey and interview data individually and in conjunction.

Results

The study yielded a nuanced portrait of the state of writing in the health sciences major. Notably, all 20 faculty members who participated in the study agreed or strongly agreed that the ability to write well is important for scholars and professionals in their field. However, the majority of participants expressed dissatisfaction or ambivalence with the state of writing in the health sciences major. Only 35% reported that their students are prepared to do the writing required in the health sciences classes they teach, and a mere 20% agreed that students who graduate with a health sciences major are adequately prepared for the writing they will do in graduate school or their professions.

Additionally, the data elucidated the context I would need to navigate as a writing center liaison. The following findings were evidenced by trends in both the survey data and interview transcripts.

Students Struggled with Discipline-Specific and Research-Related Aspects of Writing

On the survey, participants rated their average student's proficiency level in 24 writing and writing-related abilities. Although responses varied, a clear trend emerged: participants perceived their students as struggling with discipline-specific and research-related aspects of writing assignments in the major. The lowest-rated abilities (on average) were accurate citations, supporting ideas with evidence, and knowledge of disciplinary writing conventions.

Moreover, all but three participants (85%) referenced at least one aspect of students' struggles with source material in their interviews. They reported that their students struggle with finding appropriate sources, critically reading those sources, marshaling evidence to support ideas, summarizing and employing quotation effectively, synthesizing and connecting ideas, citing references in APA style, and avoiding plagiarism. The following interview excerpts reflect faculty perceptions of this struggle:

- "Getting [students] to cite correctly, and getting them to explain their author's ideas is totally foreign to them."
- "[Students] sort of lose track of what they're saying, especially if you ask them to do a literature review … They have a really hard time connecting one idea to the other."
- "They're still new [to] writing in a scientific way and knowing kind of that language."

Writing Objectives and Standards for Health Sciences Majors were Either Absent or Inconsistent

At the time of the pilot study, the strategic goals and objectives for the department that housed the health sciences major did not reference writing, although the health studies and health assessment and promotion concentrations of the major mentioned communication in their missions. None of the participants in this study said that their formal course objectives focused on writing skills, although many associated the writing tasks they assigned in their classes with the department's mission "to offer pre-professional and professional preparation for the health disciplines."

In the absence of specific writing objectives, some faculty members lacked a clear sense of where writing instruction and assessment were occurring in the health sciences curricula, as well as in general education requirements. In their interviews, 35% of participants expressed uncertainty about what writing instruction students received prior to their classes. Additionally, some participants held misconceptions about students' previous writing instruction – for example, that students are taught scientific genres and APA style in their first-year composition courses.

Moreover, in their open-ended survey responses, participants expressed a broad range of beliefs about what constitutes "good writing" in their disciplines (Appendix C). This variation, combined with the dearth of writing objectives, may help explain the widespread inconsistency in top grading considerations that participants reported in the survey. Figure 6.1 displays this lack of consensus and highlights misalignments in participants' grading priorities and writing values. The interviews confirmed this finding, as 40% of participants mentioned (and several expressed frustration with) the health sciences faculty's erratic expectations for student writing. One interview participant said, "I don't think the curriculum as a whole has a common thread of writing expectations or even writing teaching that students are getting. So I feel for students, because I do think they're getting some very mixed messages about

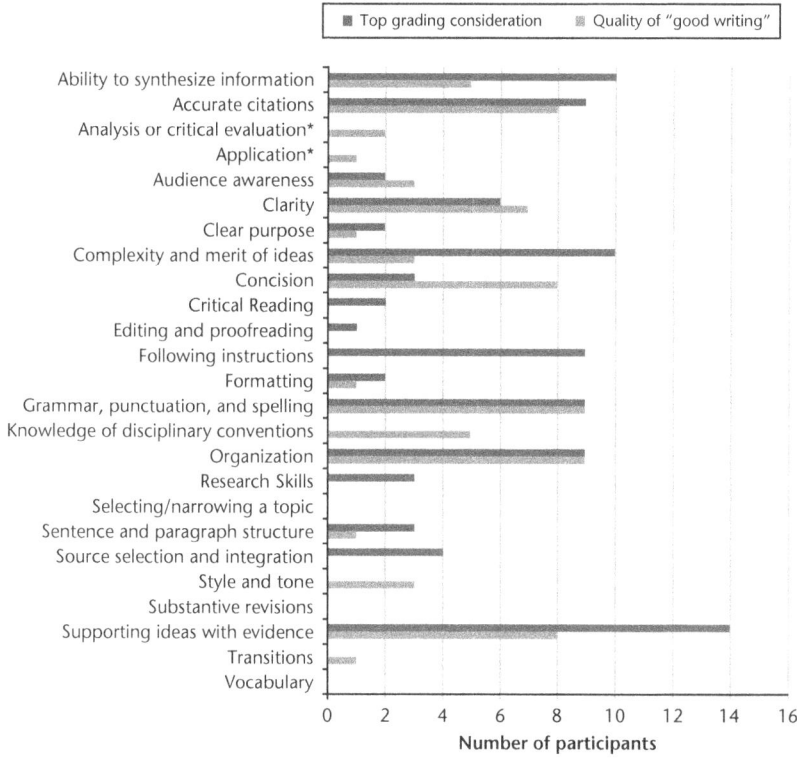

In the survey, participants listed the qualities they said characterize "good writing" in their discipline. Subsequently, they selected their five top grading considerations for writing assignments from a list of 24 writing characteristics and abilities. This figure contrasts top grading considerations with the qualities of "good writing" (derived from short-answers). Items marked with an * were associated with "good writing" but had no equivalent on the grading considerations list. Additionally, the "grammar and usage" and "punctuation and spelling" categories for top grading considerations were combined in this figure.

FIGURE 6.1   Top Grading Considerations vs. Qualities that Characterize Good Writing

what's expected in their writing … They have to figure out, 'What's the trick?', and I don't think that's what learning writing is about. That's not a fair thing to put students through, because they're figuring out professors instead of learning how to write."

Faculty Lacked Training in Writing Instruction and Feedback Strategies

In survey responses, 60% of participants agreed or strongly agreed that they feel comfortable teaching students about writing in their discipline. However, when asked what support or resources they would like to have available, more than half the participants said they wanted help with designing writing assignments, teaching writing, and/or providing feedback on writing assignments.

When asked whether they know how to provide quality feedback on writing assignments, only 50% of participants agreed or strongly agreed. More than one-third of pilot study participants reported that they feel the need to comment on every error when grading writing assignments. Additionally, in their interviews, 40% of participants indicated that they edit intensively when grading writing assignments (e.g., rewriting sentences or correcting errors in grammar, spelling, word choice, and citations). This perspective was reflected in the following interview excerpt: "I tend to get very bogged down in the nitty gritty—you know, 'this needs a comma,' 'this needs a period,' 'this is spelled wrong'—that I sometimes lose the bigger picture. So [training] would be helpful to me. I've never taken any formal professional development on how to teach writing or how to grade writing."

Administrative, Curricular, and Ideological Barriers to Writing and Writing Instruction Existed within the Major

The data illuminated several structural barriers I would need to take into account as I collaborated with faculty and administrators to develop writing interventions for health sciences majors:

> First, large class sizes and heavy teaching loads posed a significant obstacle to faculty who used (or wanted to use) writing in their courses. Within the department, the standard full-time teaching load was four classes per semester, and the average class size for participants was 44 (though some classes were as large as 150). In order to cope with these challenges, some participants said they assigned only simple writing tasks that were easy to grade, used group writing assignments to decrease the grading load, graded "content" or "ideas" only without offering feedback on writing, or gave credit for completed writing assignments without reading them. Moreover, 45% of participants said they had

changed, planned to change, or were opting not to use writing assignments because of large class sizes.

Second, at the time of the study, the health sciences major curriculum was not sequential in nature. Only a few health sciences classes had prerequisites, so students often simultaneously enrolled in courses at various levels. As a result, health sciences classes included students with a range of writing preparation and experience. This made it challenging for faculty to know what to expect of their students or how to build upon previous writing instruction.

Finally, some study participants said they believed it was not the Health Sciences faculty's responsibility to teach writing. In their survey responses, 20% of participants agreed or strongly agreed that faculty in the departments of English and Writing, Rhetoric, and Technical Communication should bear responsibility for teaching students how to write.

Discussion

While context-specific, the findings of my pilot study align with existing knowledge and theories about how students respond to writing tasks in new disciplinary contexts and about the challenges that faculty in the disciplines face when they use writing in their classes.

There is evidence that general education courses do not fully prepare students to undertake the writing required in their majors and professions (Perelman, 2011; Smith et al., 2011).

Understanding and adapting to a discipline's unique writing conventions and specialized writing tasks (or genres) proves intensely challenging for most novices (Borglin, 2012; Kilgore et al., 2013). Weiser (1999) has argued that novices are usually unaware of (and therefore apt to neglect) the following when they compose in new genres: "the structure of discourse, the level of formality, what counts as evidence, the amount of information appropriate to include for readers, whether or not to use graphics or section headings, [and] how to cite and document sources" (p. 96). Moreover, students often lack familiarity with the complex social contexts that generate writing conventions, which makes it difficult for them to anticipate the needs and expectations of their audiences (Smith et al., 2011; Zhu, 2004), an obstacle that has serious implications for their abilities to impart health literacies to their patients through tailored communication. As Jarron Slater points out in Chapter 4 of this collection, "knowing how to help someone is often not enough; helping someone also involves persuading them to act" – and rhetorical awareness (accompanied by identification with one's audience) is foundational to such acts of persuasion, enabling practitioners to understand "who [their patients] are, what they care about, and why they do the things that they do."

A number of scholars have emphasized that students learning to write in their disciplines need conventions to be explicitly explained and modeled (Autry & Carter, 2015; Elton, 2010; Smith et al., 2011). Despite this understanding, 45% of the faculty who participated in my study said they provide no writing instruction in their classes. Scholars have documented the belief that students know how (or should know how) to write before arriving in their classes among faculty who teach in pre-professional program and upper-division undergraduate courses at other institutions, particularly where students receive writing instruction in a first-year writing course (Kleinsasser et al., 1994; Smith et al, 2011). Carter (2009) has noted that faculty outside of English and composition are often unwilling to sacrifice course content to teach writing because they "conceive of writing as generalizable to all disciplines and therefore distinct from disciplinary knowledge, to be learned as a general skill outside the disciplines" (p. 385).

These barriers and misconceptions may be exacerbated by the fact that few faculty in pre-professional and professional health programs are provided formal instruction in writing pedagogy or in the complex process of scientific writing (Dankoski et al., 2012; Troxler et al., 2011) – a point that several participants in this study made in their interviews. This lack of pedagogical training, combined with the fact that many experts learn to write in their disciplines or professions through trial and error (rather than explicit instruction), means that many faculty may struggle to teach (or may even lack an awareness of) the unique features and distinctive rhetorical moves required for success in their assignments (Autry & Carter, 2015; Elton, 2010; Kilgore et al., 2013; Smith et al., 2011), including the types of written communication that health professionals employ to facilitate health literacies in patients.

Some scholars have argued that without training in how to teach writing in their disciplines, faculty may default to a "skills-based, deficit model" of teaching that focuses on fixing errors in grammar and vocabulary (Lea & Street, 1998, p. 157) instead of clarifying the connections between a discipline's ways of knowing and its writing conventions and genres (Smith et al., 2011) – a phenomenon clearly documented by this study. This "deficit model" approach is not only time consuming but also inconsistent with pedagogical best practices, which emphasize the value of formative feedback in the drafting process, the importance of prioritizing higher-order concerns, and the limited efficacy of correcting surface errors (Bean, 2011; Ferris, 2014; Haswell, 1983; Jonsson, 2013; Underwood & Tregidgo, 2006; Vardi, 2009). Even strong writers are apt to make basic errors in grammar, formatting, and logic "when faced with a particularly challenging and unfamiliar rhetorical task" (Smith et al., 2011, p. 299). Students also have a limited capacity to absorb feedback (Ferris, 2014), and when faculty focus on surface errors, they may signal that higher-order concerns (such as problems with clarity, organization, or audience awareness) are "an afterthought" (Melzer, 2014, p. 58).

As a whole, the findings of this pilot study highlighted that the health sciences major at my institution faced challenges that programs within and outside of the health professions must confront when attempting to improve students' written communication skills, particularly within disciplinary contexts. The study also offered insights into the institutional context that allowed me to identify "impact opportunities" where targeted changes within the program might broadly improve writing instruction and outcomes, namely:

- Providing tailored instruction and feedback to students engaged in discipline-specific and research-based writing;
- Developing writing objectives and consistent standards for health sciences majors; and
- Offering faculty development in writing instruction and feedback strategies.

Local Responses and Outcomes

What my colleagues and I learned through the pilot study allowed us to begin answering the question "How do we help students become better writers?" in ways that were rooted in context and empirical evidence of needs. Below are descriptions of writing initiatives and interventions that were inspired or informed by the pilot study.

Health Sciences Writing Committee

In response to the findings of the pilot study, the Health Sciences Department formed a writing committee that included faculty who teach in the major, a student in the major, a liaison librarian, and me. In its first year, the committee developed an evidence-based set of knowledge, skills, and attitudes (KSAs) for writing at each course level in the major (Appendix E). We were inspired by a set of KSAs for scholarly writing development across all levels of nursing education, which Hunker et al. (2014) developed using Bloom's Taxonomy, a model for classifying and structuring curricular learning objectives.

Acknowledging that students often take courses non-sequentially, we used our knowledge of course content and writing assignments to determine which KSAs would be appropriate for each course level. The goal of this KSA matrix was intended to serve as a first step in clarifying and aligning faculty's standards for writing assignments. I presented it to departmental faculty in the fall of 2016.

However, a number of unforeseen factors, including a departmental split, changes in leadership, faculty attrition, and changes in curriculum stalled this initiative. That said, I have used the KSA matrix informally to help faculty think about the writing they assign in their classes and to offer them vocabulary to describe writing goals and features to students.

Tailored Presentations and Workshops

In the years since I conducted the pilot study, I have provided (or, in a few cases, trained writing center tutors or other faculty members to provide) more than 75 tailored presentations and workshops in the college I serve, attended by more than 3,200 students. About a third of these events were for classes in the health sciences major, though I've found that students and faculty in across the college experience many of the same struggles as those reported in the pilot study.

The study's findings have strongly influenced my presentation topics, which often focus on features of research-heavy genres in the health sciences (e.g., scholarly introductions, literature reviews, and empirical research papers). Additionally, I've presented strategies for group writing and revision, which are especially applicable to the types of writing required of health sciences majors. These efforts also benefit faculty, who, in meeting with me to plan presentations, sometimes learn new language to describe the problems they see in student writing and ideas for how to better communicate their expectations.

Targeted Resources

Because I have limited time to offer presentations and workshops, I have sought to multiply my impact by creating online resources that address some of the most commonly cited issues in the pilot study. These are available on the writing center's website, and instructors can easily embed them in course web pages as resources or homework. Because the study emphasized students' struggles with research-based writing, I created a number of 10- to 15-minute screencasts that focus on the stylistic features of science and research writing. The most popular of those screencasts, which describes how to integrate sources into a paper written in APA style, had more than 20,200 views at the time this chapter was written. Other resources include a five-part screencast series on group writing and a video lecture and panel discussion on how to write personal statements for professional health programs. Most recently, I've created sets of resources that pair genre overviews with samples of student writing, annotated to described the writer's rhetorical moves and the paper follows (or doesn't follow) the conventions of the genre. These include overviews and samples of literature reviews, personal statements, and each section in an empirical research paper.

Faculty Development

My work in the Health Sciences Department, starting with this pilot study, has opened the door for me to regularly consult with faculty on assignment and rubric design, peer review strategies, and approaches to grading and providing feedback on writing assignments.

I have also shared writing expertise through formal faculty development workshops and resources that have reached hundreds of faculty at my university. Because half of the faculty in the pilot study reported that they do not have adequate time to provide feedback on students' writing, I offered a departmental workshop (and, later, a university-wide workshop) on write-to-learn, low-stakes, and no-grade writing assignments in spring 2017. Additionally, because the pilot study indicated that many faculty were getting bogged down by the need to comment on every error in student writing, I offered a university-wide workshop in the spring of 2018 on when to comment, what to say, and how to use rubrics when evaluating student writing. In 2019, I authored a five-part "Teaching Toolbox" series for faculty on how to effectively use peer review in their classes – a topic that often comes up when I talk to faculty about how to lighten their loads while still ensuring that students get feedback and engage in a revision process. This resource was sent to 250 faculty through my institution's Center for Faculty Innovation (CFI) and currently appears on the CFI and writing center websites.

Tutoring and Tutor Training

In addition to providing one-on-one consultations to health sciences majors, I have consistently worked to ensure that the writing center's staff of undergraduate and graduate tutors are adequately prepared to work with students composing in health disciplines. After the pilot study, the writing center changed the curriculum of its semester-long tutor training course to include the common features of research and science writing, the struggles that students have with research-based writing, and tutoring strategies that address those struggles. Tutors-in-training now practice responding to papers in common genres, such as literature reviews and personal statements.

I have also run several semester-long professional development groups for tutors on topics such as genre awareness in tutoring, tutoring literature reviews, and tutoring empirical research papers. The writing center's usage statistics suggest that these efforts are worthwhile. In the academic year following the study, 88 students came to the writing center with assignments from health sciences classes. That number increased to 130 and 112 students in the two academic years that followed. Moreover, the two writing tasks that students most frequently bring to the writing center – research papers and personal statements – frequently come from students in the health sciences major and the broader college I serve.

Honors Capstone Project Planning Course

The pilot study made clear that health sciences majors struggled with scholarly writing and that faculty felt overwhelmed by the task of giving feedback on such writing, given the many demands on their time. These issues were negatively impacting the department's honors students, who were required to conduct their honors capstone projects (almost always empirical research projects) with few formal support structures. Following the pilot study, I began offering a 3-credit honors capstone project planning course to students in the college I serve. In this course, which runs every spring, students explore the literature on their topics and, through an intensive revision process, produce formal research proposals that will guide them through their empirical research projects. This course has received excellent feedback from students and advisers alike, receiving comments on student evaluations such as "I would have had no clue where to even start with my honors project without this class" and "I feel prepared to execute a successful honors thesis, I know about the resources available to me, and I am able to critically read sources and write about them." At least one of my health sciences majors has gone on to publish her research in a scholarly journal.

If I could do anything differently, looking back, it would be to have administered a writing assessment of health sciences majors at the outset so that I could track the impact of the writing interventions and initiatives that have resulted from my study. However, I can state with confidence that students in the college I serve have more writing resources available to them and that my university's writing center is taking a much more strategic approach to serving students writing in the health and behavioral sciences. It is also worth mentioning that this study facilitated cross-disciplinary relationships in a system that tends to cloister faculty within disciplinary silos. Following the pilot study, I have engaged in interdisciplinary research projects with health sciences faculty, consulted on the creation of a new introductory course in the health sciences, and served as a judge at the Health Sciences Department's student research symposium – all arguably ways of promoting health literacies.

Limitations

The methods and instruments described in this chapter have a number of limitations. Because the survey and interview instruments were researcher-generated, additional vetting is needed to establish their reliability and validity. Self-reported data are also susceptible to measurement effects. For example, if participants had not previously considered the constructs measured by the study, the survey itself might have shaped their beliefs about and attitudes toward writing instruction and student writing. The language used in the survey and interview questions or the researcher's affiliation with the writing center could also have influenced participants' responses, creating a framing effect.

Although 45% of the faculty queried participated in the study, the study may have yielded a more complete picture of the state of writing in the health sciences major if the instruments had been designed to accommodate and elicit information from faculty who do not use writing in their classes. Additionally, if the interviews had been coded as part of a team, rather than by an individual, more trends may have emerged. Inter-coder agreement would also have increased the reliability of the analysis.

Because this study only explored faculty perspectives expressed in surveys and interviews, it did not paint a complete picture of the state of writing in the health sciences major. Follow-up studies that explore student or alumni perspectives or empirically evaluate writing samples could enrich findings. Finally, while the specific results of the pilot study may have applications to other programs in the health professions or writing centers, they are not generalizable, given their local nature.

Conclusion

In professional and pre-professional health programs, students' writing abilities affect not only their academic success but also their prospects and efficacy as health professionals (Gopee & Deane, 2013; Schryer & Spoel, 2005).

In particular, they must prepare to use written communication to help their patients evaluate risks, prevent adverse outcomes, understand diagnoses, and make informed treatment decisions (HHS, 2010). Their patients' health literacies may depend, for example, upon their ability to translate highly technical research studies into accessible, actionable information – or their willingness to create or revise existing resources to take into account the needs and identities of their audiences.

There is, however, no one-size-fits-all intervention that will ensure students develop as writers, as every program is part of an intricate system that shapes its particular needs, strengths, problems, constraints, and resources. The best writing interventions and initiatives will account for this complex network of variables by employing the principles of evidence-based practice: first, programs should map the systems they operate within so that they can accurately diagnose writing-related needs and problems; then, they can respond with interventions that integrate research, local expertise, and the values and preferences of students and faculty. The instruments I created for this study can help facilitate that process – not only within programs preparing students to enter health professions but also within those preparing students to enter other fields.

Instructors and program administrators who are interested in using this approach to better understand the state of writing in their contexts might also consider the following:

- Cross-disciplinary collaborations might be a useful option for those with limited time and resources to dedicate to institutional research. Administrators and faculty in academic and pre-professional programs, campus writing program administrators, composition faculty, writing center administrators, and liaison librarians may have uses for the data generated by this model and may, therefore, be willing to help with data collection and analysis.

- I recommend having someone from outside of the program being studied conduct interviews, as participants could be more inclined to speak candidly with outsiders.
- The survey and interview instruments I created for this study can be used individually, customized, or curtailed for a less demanding research experience.
- The instruments used in this study could be adapted for use among students, who may verify, challenge, or enrich faculty perspectives.
- Ideally, interventions that programs develop in response to problems revealed by the instruments should be assessed via pre- and post-intervention studies. Qualitative assessments of writing samples, while time consuming, may produce the richest data.

I hope that the tools and experiences shared in this chapter will empower other faculty and administrators to strategically approach writing instruction, writing interventions, and writing assessments in their programs. I also hope that they will contribute to efforts to train health professionals, and others, who are not only health literate but also capable of facilitating health literacies in their patients and through their organizations.

References

Autry, M. K., & Carter, M. (2015). Unblocking occluded genres in graduate writing: Thesis and dissertation support services at North Carolina State University. *Composition Forum*, 31. https://files.eric.ed.gov/fulltext/EJ1061566.pdf

Bean, J. C. (2011). *Engaging ideas: The professor's guide to integrating writing, critical thinking, and active learning in the classroom* (2nd ed.) Jossey-Bass.

Borglin, G. (2012). Promoting critical thinking and academic writing skills in nurse education. *Nurse Education Today*, 32(5), 611–613. 10.1016/j.nedt.2011.06.009

Carter, S. (2009). The writing center paradox: Talk about legitimacy and the problem of institutional change. *College Composition and Communication*, 61(1), 133–152.

Dankoski, M. E., Palmer, M. M., Banks, J., Brutkiewicz, R. R., Walvoord, E. C., Longtin, K., Bogdewic, S., & Gopen, G. D. (2012). Academic writing: Supporting faculty in a critical competency for success. *Journal of Faculty Development*, 26(2), 47–54.

Duke, C. R. (1982). Survey of writing in various disciplines. Murray State University. https://files.eric.ed.gov/fulltext/ED232167.pdf

Elton, L. (2010). Academic writing and tacit knowledge. *Teaching in Higher Education*, 15(2), 151–160. 10.1080/13562511003619979

Epstein, M. H. (1999). Teaching field-specific writing: Results of a WAC survey. *Business and Professional Communication Quarterly*, 62(1), 29–38. 10.1177%2F108056999906200103

Ferris, D. R. (2014). Responding to student writing: Teachers' philosophies and practices. *Assessing Writing*, 19, 6–23. 10.1016/j.asw.2013.09.004

Gopee, N., & Deane, M. (2013). Strategies for successful academic writing — institutional and non-institutional support for students. *Nurse Education Today*, 33(12), 1624–1631. 10.1016/j.nedt.2013.02.004

Haswell, R. H. (1983). Minimal marking. *College English*, 45(6), 600–604. 10.2307/377147

Hunker, D. F., Gazza, E. A., & Shellenbarger, T. (2014). Evidence-based knowledge, skills, and attitudes for scholarly writing development across all levels of nursing education. *Journal of Professional Nursing*, 30(4), 341–346. 10.1016/j.profnurs.2013.11.003

Jonsson, A. (2013). Facilitating productive use of feedback in higher education. *Active Learning in Higher Education*, 14(1), 63–76. 10.1177%2F1469787412467125

Kilgore, C. D., Cronley, C., & Amey, B. (2013). Developing grass roots writing resources: A novel approach to writing within the social work discipline. *Teaching in Higher Education*, 18(8), 920–932. 10.1080/13562517.2013.827647

Kleinsasser, A. M., Collins, N. D., & Nelson, J. (1994). Writing in the disciplines: Teacher as gatekeeper and as border crosser. *Journal of General Education*, 43(2), 117–133.

Lea M. R., & Street B. V. (1998). Student writing in higher education: An academic literacies approach. *Studies in Higher Education*, 23(2), 157–172. 10.1080/03075 079812331380364

Mackenzie, S. (2018). Writing for public health: Strategies for teaching writing in a school or program of public health. *Public Health Reports*, 133(5), 614–618. 10.1177/0033354 918785374

Maimon, E. P., & Nodine, B. F. (1978, December). Measuring behavior and attitude in the teaching of writing among faculties in various disciplines [Conference paper presentation]. 93rd Annual Meeting of the Modern Language Association of America, New York, NY.

Melzer, D. (2014). *Assignments across the curriculum: A national study of college writing*. Utah State University Press.

Melzer, D. (2013). Using systems thinking to transform writing programs. *WPA: Writing Program Administration*, 36(2), 75–94.

Oermann, M. H., Leonardelli, A. K., Turner, K. M., Hawks, S. J., Derouin, A. L., & Hueckel, R. M. (2015). Systematic review of educational programs and strategies for developing students' and nurses' writing skills. *Journal of Nursing Education*, 54(1), 28–34. 10.3928/01484834-20141224-01

Pasewaldt, S. E., Baller, S. L., Blackstone, S., & Bryan Malenke, L. Impact of a hand hygiene curriculum and group handwashing station at two primary schools in east Africa. *International Quarterly of Community Health Education*, 39(3), 175–187. 10.1177%2F0272684X18819968

Perelman, L. (2011, December). WAC revisited: You get what you pay for. *The Writing Instructor*. https://files.eric.ed.gov/fulltext/EJ959704.pdf

Schryer C. F., & Spoel, P. (2005). Genre theory, health-care discourse, and professional identity formation. *Journal of Business and Technical Communication*, 19(3), 249–278. 10.1177/F1050651905275625

Smith, T. G., Ariail, J., Richards-Slaughter, S., & Kerr, L. (2011). Teaching professional writing in an academic health sciences center: The writing center model at the Medical University of South Carolina. *Teaching and Learning in Medicine*, 23(3), 298–300. 10.1080/10401334.2011.586937

Troxler, H., Jacobson Vann, J. C., & Oermann, M. H. (2011). How baccalaureate nursing programs teach writing. *Nursing Forum*, 46(4), 280–288. 10.1111/j.1744-6198.2011. 00242.x

Underwood, J. S., & Tregidgo, A. P. (2006). Improving student writing through effective feedback: Best practices and recommendations. *Journal of Teaching Writing*, 22(2), 73–97. http://journals.iupui.edu/index.php/teachingwriting/article/view/1346/1295

U.S. Department of Health and Human Services, Office of Disease Prevention and Health Promotion. (2010). *National action plan to improve health literacy*. https://health.gov/sites/default/files/2019-09/Health_Literacy_Action_Plan.pdf

Vardi, I. (2009). The relationship between feedback and change in tertiary student writing in the disciplines. *International Journal of Teaching and Learning in Higher Education*, 20(3), 350–361. https://files.eric.ed.gov/fulltext/EJ869319.pdf

Weiser, I. (1999). Local research and curriculum development: Using surveys to learn about writing in the disciplines. In I. Weiser & S. K. Rose (Eds.), *The writing program administrator as researcher: Inquiry in action & reflection* (pp. 95–103). Heinemann.

Zerger, S. (1997, March 13). "This is chemistry, not literature": Faculty perceptions of student writing [Conference paper presentation]. 48th Annual Meeting of the Conference on College Composition and Communication, Phoenix, AZ. http://files.eric.ed.gov/fulltext/ED411515.pdf

Zhu, W. (2004). Faculty views on the importance of writing, the nature of academic writing, and teaching and responding to writing in the disciplines. *Journal of Second Language Writing*, 13(1), 29–48. 10.1016/j.jslw.2004.04.004

Appendix A: Faculty Survey Questions

1. Name (fill in the blank)
2. Please list each course you are currently teaching or have taught in the Health Sciences major in the past year (summer 2014, fall 2015, or spring 2015). For each course, note approximately how many typed, double-spaced pages students complete for **individual** writing assignments and how many typed, double-spaced pages students complete for **group** writing assignments.

	Course Prefix and Number	Typed, double-spaced pages required for **individual** writing assignments	Typed, double-spaced pages required for **group** writing assignments
Course 1			
Course 2			
Course 3			
Course 4			
Course 5			
Course 6			
Course 7			

3. Which of the following writing assignments and tasks do you use in your classes?

- Personal reflection papers
- Book or article reviews/responses
- Annotated bibliographies
- Literature reviews
- Research papers
- Lab reports
- Argument/position papers
- Critical/analytical essays
- Essay questions on tests or exams
- Observation logs
- Online discussion boards
- Blogs
- Journals
- Ungraded in-class or out-of-class writing as a lead-in to class discussion
- Other _____

4. In your discipline, what qualities characterize good writing? (open-ended)
5. Do you require students to complete multiple drafts of major writing assignments? (yes/no)
6. Do students receive writing instruction in your classes? (yes/no)
7. In general, do you feel that your students are prepared to do the writing required of them in your classes? (yes/no)
8. What is your average student's proficiency level for the following writing and writing-related abilities: (poor, fair, good, excellent, not sure, not applicable)

- Organization
- Selecting/narrowing a topic
- Complexity and merit of ideas
- Clear purpose
- Awareness of audience
- Following assignment instructions
- Research skills
- Supporting ideas with evidence
- Appropriate selection and integration of source material
- Accurate citations
- Knowledge of disciplinary writing conventions
- Ability to synthesize information and ideas
- Clarity
- Style and tone
- Concision

- Formatting
- Sentence and paragraph structure
- Transitions
- Vocabulary
- Grammar and usage
- Punctuation and spelling
- Making substantive revisions
- Editing and proofreading

9. Of the writing and writing-related abilities that you saw in the previous question, please select and rank the **top five** that you take into consideration **when grading** writing assignments (1 being the most important):

- Organization
- Selecting/narrowing a topic
- Complexity and merit of ideas
- Clear purpose
- Awareness of audience
- Following assignment instructions
- Research skills
- Supporting ideas with evidence
- Appropriate selection and integration of source material
- Accurate citations
- Knowledge of disciplinary writing conventions
- Ability to synthesize information and ideas
- Clarity
- Style and tone
- Concision
- Formatting
- Sentence and paragraph structure
- Transitions
- Vocabulary
- Grammar and usage
- Punctuation and spelling
- Making substantive revisions
- Editing and proofreading

10. Approximately what percentage of your students' overall grades in your courses is based on writing assignments? (open-ended)
11. Which of the following do you offer your students:

- Consultations about writing or writing assignments (during class or office hours)
- In-class peer review sessions

- Written feedback (from the instructor) on paper ideas and/or thesis statements
- Written feedback on rough drafts
- Scored rubrics for final drafts
- Written sentence/paragraph level feedback on final drafts
- Written global/overall feedback on final drafts
- The opportunity to revise a paper after receiving a grade

12. Please indicate your opinions of the following statements:
(strongly disagree, disagree, neither agree nor disagree, agree, strongly agree, not sure)

- Writing is a good tool for assessing a students' acquisition of knowledge.
- Writing assignments help students learn.
- Writing assignments encourage critical thinking.
- The ideas in a paper are more important than the way it is written.
- My students are generally invested and interested in their writing assignments.
- I talk to my students about my own writing and writing process.
- I feel comfortable teaching students about writing in my discipline.
- I am confident in my ability to design writing assignments.
- I feel like I have adequate time to provide feedback on my students' writing assignments.
- I know how to provide quality feedback on writing assignments.
- When grading papers, I feel the need to comment on every error.
- Writing instruction should be the responsibility of faculty in the departments of English and Writing, Rhetoric, and Technical Communication.
- Students should be required to do more writing as part of the Health Sciences major.
- Students who graduate with a Health Sciences major are adequately prepared for the writing they will do in graduate school or in their professions.
- The ability to write well is important for scholars and professionals in my field.
- I feel confident about my writing ability.
- I enjoy writing.

13. Please answer the following questions: (yes/no/not sure)

- I know what services the University Writing Center offers students and faculty.
- I have encouraged students to visit the University Writing Center.
- My students have visited the University Writing Center.

- I have invited the University Writing Center to give a presentation or workshop in my class(es).
- I have had a one-on-one consultation with a University Writing Center faculty member.

14. How many years have you been teaching college level classes in the field of health sciences?

- 0–1
- 1–5
- 5–10
- 10–15
- 15–20
- 20–25
- more than 25

Appendix B: Faculty Interview Questions

1. Based on your experience and observations, how would you describe the state of writing in the Health Sciences major?
2. What evidence, if any, have you observed that students are using writing skills they've been taught in earlier classes—either general education or Health Sciences classes?
3. What are the biggest challenges your students face, when it comes to academic writing? What are the barriers to their success as academic writers?
4. Would you give me a brief overview of the major writing assignments you use in your classes? Also, could you explain what the purpose, or learning objectives, of those assignments are, and how they connect to the broader learning objectives for the course?
5. Do you think students are achieving those objectives through their writing assignments? (If necessary, follow up: What's working? What's not going as planned?)
6. [If faculty member uses group assignments] How do you prepare students for the challenges of writing in groups?
7. What strategies and resources do you use, if any, to help your students improve as writers?
8. Have you observed students improving as writers—either over the course of your class, or over the course of the major? Explain. (Follow-up: What do you think is helping them improve? OR Why do you think they aren't improving)
9. [If faculty member encourages students to visit Writing Center] What are you hoping they will get out of their visit to the University Writing Center? Have you noticed any improvement in the writing of students who visit the Writing Center?
10. What kind of support or resources would you like to have available to you, in regards to your own writing or teaching writing to your students?

Appendix C: Coding Categories for Survey Question 4 (Table 6.1)

TABLE 6.1 Coding Categories for Survey Question 4[a]

Writing Ability Category	Number of references
Analysis or critical evaluation	2
Application	1
Audience or context awareness	3
Awareness of disciplinary or genre conventions	6
Citations and APA style	8
Clarity	7
Complexity, originality, or merit of ideas	3
Concision	9
Format	1
Grammar, punctuation, or spelling	11
Organization, structure, and flow	9
Purpose	2
Sentence and paragraph structure	1
Style and voice	1
Supporting ideas with evidence	8
Synthesis of information and ideas	5
Transitions	**1**

Note

a Participants provided open-ended responses to the question, "In your discipline, what qualities characterize good writing?" This table shows the writing ability categories into which responses were placed, as well as the number of references each category received.

Appendix D: Themes and subthemes used in qualitative analysis of interviews (Table 6.2)

TABLE 6.2 Themes and Subthemes Used in Qualitative Analysis of Interviews

Themes and subthemes	Number of sources (aggregated)	Number of references (aggregated)
Faculty attitudes	20	384
Expressions of emotion about teaching	12	26
References to student attitudes, writing, and ability	20	309
Mixed	19	56
Negative	20	157
Neutral	12	29
Positive	18	67

(*Continued*)

TABLE 6.2 (Continued)

Themes and subthemes	Number of sources (aggregated)	Number of references (aggregated)
References to other faculty (impact on state of writing)	9	30
Mixed	3	3
Negative	8	19
Neutral	3	3
Positive	2	5
References to their own writing	6	12
Taking responsibility for writing-related problems	5	7
Observed problems in student writing	20	215
Grammar, spelling, mechanics	11	23
Informal, conversational, or text-like writing	5	9
Lack of clarity	4	8
Lack of transfer from previous classes	6	9
Not following instructions	4	6
Polishing, editing, or formatting issues	7	12
Problems with source material	17	88
Citations and APA	10	29
Critical reading	4	8
Finding appropriate sources	7	11
Inability to summarize	2	3
Not enough evidence to support ideas	3	3
Plagiarism	4	10
Problems synthesizing and connecting ideas	6	14
Relying too much on summary or copy and paste	7	9
Structure and organization	10	16
Transitions	2	2
Underdeveloped ideas	7	8
Unfamiliarity with conventions (academic, discipline-specific, genre)	12	28
Wordiness or lack of focus	1	3
Observed student attitudes and mindsets (problematic)	19	106
Attitudes toward education	13	28
Banking model or "regurgative" style of learning	2	3
Dependence or wanting things handed to them	7	14
Fixation on grades	4	6
Unwillingness to seek help	2	2

(Continued)

TABLE 6.2 (Continued)

Themes and subthemes	Number of sources (aggregated)	Number of references (aggregated)
Attitudes toward writing	7	21
Equating time spent with quality of product	2	2
Lack of confidence	3	4
Not perceiving writing as a process that takes time	5	7
Not perceiving writing as essential to their discipline	4	6
Lifestyle or general	17	56
Defensiveness	3	5
Distracted	4	5
Fear of failure	1	1
Lack of motivation or initiative, not care or trying	9	22
Problems with time management	7	11
Problems working in groups	10	12
Potential threats/barriers to success	19	192
Challenges posed by group work	4	4
Complaining (amongst faculty) about student writing	2	2
Curricular problems	3	3
Challenges teaching English Language Learners	6	6
Expectations and standards for students	16	41
Inconsistency among faculty	8	12
Other faculty are too lenient	2	6
Other faculty are too stringent	3	4
Incorrect assumptions about previous instruction	4	5
Students not fulfilling faculty expectations	8	10
Uncertainty about expectations and standards	2	2
Uncertainty about prior writing instruction that students receive	7	12
Potentially problematic grading strategies	14	26
Intensive editing	8	16
Only grading content or ideas	7	8
Large class sizes	13	34
Changing, planning to change, or not using writing assignments as a result of class size	9	17
Giving grading to graduate or teaching assistants	1	2

(Continued)

TABLE 6.2 (Continued)

Themes and subthemes	Number of sources (aggregated)	Number of references (aggregated)
Not grading writing assignments	4	5
Using group work to manage grading load	5	6
Pressure of covering a lot of content	7	13
Responsibility for writing instruction	13	29
References to grade school and previous education	8	16
Who should be responsible for teaching writing	11	13
Students don't know what APA is	4	4
Students not held accountable	1	2
Teachers not caring about writing	1	1
Potentially problematic ideas about fairness	1	3
Research, writing, or thinking as process	13	30
Teaching practices and strategies	20	215
Adapting assignments based on experiences or feedback	10	17
Building group dynamics	10	22
Group consultations or mediation	2	2
Instruction on group dynamics/teamwork	5	5
Teambuilding activities	4	4
Writing instruction	6	8
Flexibility with students	5	6
Formal assessment of writing assignment efficacy	1	2
Instruction on research practices	3	4
Office hour consultations	13	27
Other	2	2
Outside resources an initiatives	19	55
Madison Collaborative / 8 Key Questions for ethical reasoning	3	3
Center for Instructional Technology or Center for Faculty Innovation	2	2
Libraries	10	12
Links, guides, and other resources	7	12
University Writing Center	18	25
Peer evaluations for team based writing assignments	4	4
Peer reviews	4	6
Providing sample assignments or templates	6	8
Rubrics for writing assignments	10	18
	6	7

(Continued)

TABLE 6.2 (Continued)

Themes and subthemes	Number of sources (aggregated)	Number of references (aggregated)
Scaffolding writing assignments or multiple drafts		
Specific writing assignment criteria	9	12
Written feedback on writing assignments	12	16
University Writing Center	20	106
Misconceptions about the UWC	8	8
References to UWC Liaison to CHBS	4	8
Attitudes toward UWC	18	44
Negative	2	2
Neutral/Uncertain	6	7
Positive	15	35
Areas students need help with when visiting UWC		
English language learner issues	2	2
Higher order/global concerns	7	19
Genre Awareness	3	4
Organization	4	7
Synthesis or integrating sources	3	8
Later order concerns	13	22
Citations	5	6
Concision	2	2
Proofreading (grammar, spelling, etc.)	6	7
Style	5	5
Transitions	2	2
The writing process	7	8
Ideas and suggestions for UWC	8	8
Concerns about UWC tutoring services	3	5
Utility of writing assignments and instruction	20	218
Assignment purposes and goals (skills/ knowledge developed or used)	20	155
Audience awareness	3	4
Concision	3	3
Critical reading	5	7
Employing disciplinary conventions	9	19
Finding and/or integrating research	14	20
Following instructions	1	2
Forming or supporting opinions with evidence	8	17
Fostering critical thinking or critical evaluation	16	32
Learning, applying, or engaging course materials	14	38
Self-reflection	4	10

(Continued)

TABLE 6.2 (Continued)

Themes and subthemes	Number of sources (aggregated)	Number of references (aggregated)
Teamwork	2	3
Future applications	18	62
Applications in jobs or field	14	27
Helping to develop complex view of healthcare system, society, or world	8	14
Learning to work with others	6	7
Preparing students for graduate school	8	13
Learning assessment	1	1
What students like and dislike	12	21
Dislike	8	10
Like	4	10
What's working vs. what's not working	7	11
Strategies for teaching writing that are not working	3	3
Strategies for teaching writing that are not working	5	8

The researcher developed a list of themes while transcribing interviews and then developed and refined those themes during qualitative analysis. The themes and subthemes in this table were entered and used as nodes in NVivo9. The themes highlighted in gray represent parent nodes, and nodes below them are indented to indicate level of sub-theme. Column 2 shows the number of sources (or participants) employed a theme at least once. Column 3 shows the total number of times a theme or subtheme was referenced in the entire body of interviews. The numbers in both columns represent aggregates (parent nodes include all sub-nodes). In some cases, references were coded only at a parent node. Additionally, many references were coded at multiple nodes.

Appendix E: Knowledge, Skills, and Attitudes for Writing in the Health Sciences Major (Table 6.3)

TABLE 6.3 Knowledge, Skills, and Attitudes for Writing in the Health Sciences Major, Arranged by Course Level

	Knowledge	Skills	Attitudes
100-level	Recognizes the roles that summarizing, paraphrasing, and quotation play academic writing	Performs prewriting activities (such as freewriting, cluster mapping, and outlining) to facilitate writing[a]	Perceives writing as a process, not merely a product

(Continued)

TABLE 6.3 (Continued)

	Knowledge	Skills	Attitudes
	Knows what services and resources exist on campus to provide writing support (e.g., the University Writing Center, professors' office hours, and subject librarians)	Identifies and describes key ideas in scholarly and scientific articles, using one's own words	Values and reads instructor feedback on writing assignments
	Recognizes the function of common features of APA guidelines (such as formatting and citations)	Identifies common errors in grammar, mechanics, and formatting in written work	
	Knows what constitutes plagiarism	Considers the audience and purpose of types of writing assigned and encountered in Health Sciences classes	
		Demonstrates professionalism in written communications with instructors and/or peers (e.g., emails or discussion boards)	
200-level	Recognizes common features of scholarly and scientific writing in the Health Sciences (e.g., concision, objectivity, formal language, formatting guidelines)	Drafts, reviews, and revises written work before submitting it	Believes that writing is a skill that can be improved, not an innate ability
	Recognizes the functions of written communication in the health professions	Paraphrases scholarly and scientific writing using original wording, sentence structure, and style	Values opportunities to participate in peer review (both as a reviewer and a writer)

(*Continued*)

TABLE 6.3 (Continued)

Knowledge	Skills	Attitudes
	Organizes writing logically	Acknowledges the attitudes and emotions one associates with writing[a]
	Generally follows grammar rules and formatting guidelines in written work	
	Follows APA guidelines when citing sources and building reference lists	
	Reviews written work for plagiarism and properly attributes sources	
	Uses instructor and/or peer feedback to improve writing[a]	
	Uses appropriate services and resources to develop writing skills (e.g., campus services, relevant websites, or style guides)	
	Effectively employs terminology introduced in the course	
	Contributes to team-based writing assignments	
	Develops strategies for collaborative writing and revising	
	Budgets appropriate time for writing tasks and completes writing assignments over multiple sessions	

(*Continued*)

TABLE 6.3 (Continued)

	Knowledge	Skills	Attitudes
300-level	Differentiates the characteristics of various academic writing tasks and genres (e.g., reflection papers, critical analyses, and research papers)	Demonstrates critical thinking and/or application of course content in writing	Selects strategies to manage the emotional aspects of writing[b]
	Recognizes audiences and purposes of academic and professional writing tasks in the Health Sciences	Engages in substantive revision of writing (e.g., reorganizing, developing ideas, or resolving gaps and inconsistencies)	Values the role of written communication in providing tailored and effective care to patients or clients
		Produces accurate summaries of scholarly articles using one's own words[a]	Values the connection between scholarly writing and evidence-based practice[a]
		Writes in accordance with the expectations of the genre or writing task	
		Achieves intended purpose in written work (e.g., persuades, informs, analyzes, or critiques)	
		Uses language and style appropriate for assigned writing tasks	
		Effectively manages the challenges of writing in teams	
		Identifies and seeks to address long-term patterns of error or problems in writing (e.g., consistent comma errors, lack of transitions between ideas, or weak conclusions)	

(*Continued*)

TABLE 6.3 (Continued)

	Knowledge	Skills	Attitudes
400–level	Recognizes writing strategies used by scholars and professionals in the Health Sciences	Produces writing in scholarly and/or professional genres (e.g., journal articles, case studies, literature reviews, or proposals)[a] Produces persuasive and polished career development documents (e.g., personal statement, cover letter, resume, or professional philosophy) Demonstrates adherence to the ethical principles of writing[b] Synthesizes information from multiple sources to generate new insights, provide context for research, or make recommendations for evidence-based practice Submits writing that is virtually free of surface-level errors Identifies audience and tailors written communication for a variety of audiences (scholars, health providers, general public, etc.) Demonstrates proficiency in using APA guidelines and scholarly writing conventions	Seeks out mentorship in writing and scholarly development[a]

Notes

a   These KSA were adapted from Hunker et al.'s (2014) "KSAs by Nursing Education Level"

b   These KSA were directly quoted from Hunker et al.'s (2014) "KSAs by Nursing Education Level"

7

REFLECTION FOR HEALTH LITERACIES IN THE HEALTH SCIENCE CURRICULUM

Yuko Taniguchi, Aaron Bruenger, Bronson Lemer, and Jennifer Wacek

At the time of graduation, students are equipped to attend to complex problems in society as well as the unknown and unpredictable problems that will arise in the future. Such a grand mission for higher education seems hefty today as the world has navigated unpredictable problems during the COVID-19 pandemic. Searching for solutions, exploring options, processing information, and sharing knowledge while tolerating pressure, stress, and ambiguity has been the experience of current healthcare workers. Students in the fields of Medicine and Health Sciences are expected to acquire a unique set of abilities and attributes beyond academic knowledge and practical skills in order to combat work stress and ambiguity. With this expectation, educators increasingly shift their focus to the holistic development of learners by bringing awareness to health literacies. As defined by Sorensen et al. (2012), health literacy refers to:

> people's knowledge, motivation, and competences to access, understand, appraise and apply health information in order to make judgments and take decisions in everyday life concerning healthcare, disease prevention and health promotion to maintain or improve quality of life during the life course.

What practices effectively engage students to encompass the necessary dimensions of learning to strengthen their health literacies, thus becoming promoters of health literacies in the healthcare workforce?

Reflection is a critical skill and practice contributing to health literacies, as other contributors to this collection have already described. Learning encompasses three dimensions: cognitive (gaining knowledge and skills), emotional (balancing mental energy, feelings, and motivation to develop sensitivity), and social (communicating

DOI: 10.4324/9781003316770-10

and cooperating through external interactions) (Illeris, 2002). Intentional reflective practice requires utilizing all three dimensions, allowing a critical examination of various components that contribute to high health literacies.

Reflective practice in the health science curriculum is commonly found in writing. Wald et al. (2015) argue that reflective writing provides students the opportunity to develop the important metacognition and emotional awareness that is necessary for them to develop a professional identity that reflects the values and complexity of the profession. Health programs have used reflective writing as a tool to realize strategies for connecting with patients and their families and to recognize an appreciation for diverse social groups (Kerr, 2010). In addition, students gain appreciation and positive attitudes and outlooks regarding future challenges by reflecting on the past challenges they have navigated (Koh et al., 2014). Reflective practice has been found as an effective means of developing the observational and evaluative skills necessary for future health practitioners.

Despite the recognition of reflective practice, it is rarely integrated as an essential component of health education programs. Many programs treat reflective practice as supplemental to the science-based curriculum that is considered the core of health education (Locher, 2017; Sandars, 2009). Compounding this problem is the tendency to conflate reflective writing with creative writing, which may devalue it in programs where the perceived objectivity of scientific data is valued (Kerr, 2010). In addition, both reflective and creative writing is included under the justification of medical humanities or narrative medicine (Kerr, 2010). Although these fields have growing respect in medical education, they are not viewed as essential fields of medical knowledge, the way that anatomy, immunology, or organic chemistry are. While the focus on scientific knowledge has traditionally been a critical component of health science education, it represents a shortcoming in addressing the needs of contemporary students. Considering the abilities undergraduate students are asked to gain to be ready for the uncertainty of the 21st century, *centering* reflective practice is a necessary step. (See also Chapter 3 and Chapter 4.)

In the process of including reflective practice to a valued place, it is crucial for educators to understand how and why learning, as well as non-learning, occurs. Illeris (2004) provides insightful explanations on the obstacles to intended learning as he incorporates the types of learnings identified by a psychologist, Thomas Nissen (1970, as cited in Illeris, 2004) and transformative learning theory defined by Jack Mezirow (1981, 1992, 1997). Illeris argues that learning requires cognitive, emotional, and social dimensions.

In the cognitive dimension, the obstacle is generally seen in the absence of necessary knowledge and skills. For example, Nissen (1970, as cited in Illeris, 2004) describes two types of learning: *cumulation*, in which a learner learns through a type of mechanical learning, and *assimilation,* in which a learner adds new insights and meaning to knowledge that is previously established. Knowledge gained from cumulation and assimilation are applied in situations that are similar to the original learning context and environment. A learner, who is unable to gain knowledge in the cognitive dimension, is likely to have arrived with not enough prior knowledge, skills, and experiences to comprehend new information.

In the emotional dimension, the obstacle is seen in mental defense. For example, Nissen (1970, as cited in Illeris, 2004) describes a type of learning, *accommodation,* in which learners break down their previous understanding and reconstruct it as the new situation calls for this evaluation. This process of learning is often painful for learners. Yet, once processed, their new understanding can be utilized in the context different from the original learning context and environment (Illeris, 2004).

In the social dimension, the obstacle is closely tied to resistance in the emotional dimension. A learner actively resists a certain type of learning structure that is presented to them (Mezirow, 1992). For example, a learner may reject a certain social structure, firmly believing that the system itself is flawed. This resistance may come across as frustrating to educators, yet Illeris (2003, 2004) states that this sort of active resistance can be crucial for non-learning to turn into learning.

Resistance is an opportunity for a turning point according to Mezirow's Transformative Theory, which articulates that a learner shifts their point of view at a critical moment when they can no longer resist. Each learner holds a certain habitual way of thinking that develops into assumptions. Mezirow (1997) calls this, "frame of reference" (pp.5). A learner is called to transform their frame of reference when they encounter an unavoidable situation that challenges their assumption and their habitual way of thinking can no longer make sense of their situation. Navigating such a crisis-like situation provides doubts and a strong "identity defense," as students feel as if their identity is threatened (Illeris, 2004). Simultaneously, a learner is forced to engage in critical self-reflection. It is in this space of being critical and reflective that a learner becomes aware of not only their own point of view, bias, and judgments, but also what surrounds them: cultural, social, and political views developed by others. With this awareness of self, others, and the larger context of the world, a learner begins to reconstruct their cognitive, emotional, and social dimensions of learning.

Upon processing and accepting the insights that emerge from reflection, a learner is able to take action. Mezirow (1991) articulates that "all transformative learning involves taking action to implement insights derived from critical re-flection" (p. 225). In other words, the evidence of one's transformation is beyond gaining insights; it requires one to have changed, which can be seen through changes in behavior. Transformative learning theory is especially relevant to undergraduate students who are met with various situations that will challenge all three dimensions of learning. It means that this learning period contains the strong potential for students to transform their learning. Having reflective practice as the central component of college education, students can practice how to face their own resistance in a structured and supportive environment.

The centering of reflective writing requires educators to first become aware of obstacles within each dimension and develop an effective reflective practice that maximizes students' learning. The intentionality of reflective practice is critical in connecting to learning. Thus, gaining the benefits of reflective writing requires structure and guidance (Sandars, 2009). Simply asking students to reflect on a situation will not result in positive outcomes. Students must be provided a structure that allows for in depth reflection, tools that allow them to move beyond the more obvious aspects of their experience, and guidance that "supportively challenges" (Sandars, 2009) their assumptions. This requires thoughtful implementation on the part of the faculty. An additional complication is that reflective writing, especially as it is used in health education, is not a clearly defined genre. As Locher (2017) points out, reflective writing can take many forms, from prose narratives and scripts, to more expository and analytical writing, to even bulleted lists. Jarron Slater described some of these forms in Chapter 4 of this collection. With such varying structural differences, it can be hard to ensure that health students engage in the sustained act of guided reflection that will effectively challenge them in ways that result in their emotional, cognitive, and social growth.

Case Study: Reflective Writing Curriculum, Bachelor of Science in Health Sciences at the University of Minnesota Rochester

We present the reflective writing curriculum of the Bachelor of Science in Health Sciences (BSHS) program at the University of Minnesota Rochester (UMR) as a case study in which reflection is cultivated as an essential part of Health Sciences education and celebrated as a community value, one that is as crucial to students' learning as biological knowledge or quantitative reasoning. Reflection has become a part of the culture of UMR, thus the provision of resources meaningfully reflects the motivation to engage in the practice and is supported by the entire community. (In Chapter 6, Lucy Bryan Malenke details another health science program, at James Madison University.)

UMR is the most recent campus in the University of Minnesota system. It is a small campus of fewer than 1,000 undergraduate students and whose faculty focus on educational innovation. The primary educational program is its Bachelor of Science in Health Sciences, an interdisciplinary program that provides students foundational knowledge for going into a variety of health careers. There is only one academic unit at UMR, the Center for Learning Innovation (CLI), composed of faculty in the sciences, the social sciences, and the humanities. The interdisciplinary nature of the department and the program has allowed us to scaffold the teaching of reflective writing throughout the curriculum. It has also opened up opportunities to implement reflective writing instruction into other disciplinary courses. This way students receive consistent instruction and models for reflective writing that supportively challenge the students as they make their way through their undergraduate education.

Integrating our multiyear reflective writing curriculum into the coursework of the BSHS program has required a recognition of the importance of reflective practice for our students. It is a practice that has been supported by our administrators, as well as our colleagues who teach in other disciplines. Explicit reflective writing instruction occurs in five small-credit, writing-focused courses, all of which are requirements for the program, as well as having guided reflective writing assignments incorporated in a number of courses in other disciplines. In addition, final reflection assignments, a reflective essay, and a presentation based on the essay, are crucial parts of each student's Capstone that is required for graduation. In order to support this process, we have five writing faculty, one committee composed of ten faculty from a variety of disciplines, 32 faculty members to serve as Capstone advisors that evaluate the final reflections, one administrative assistant, and the regular support of one IT staff member.

Reflection Models

Two primary models utilized in the multiyear reflection curriculum in UMR are the ABCs of Reflection Writing and ABCs123 Reflective Writing model. The first model was informed by the work of Hondagneu-Sotelo and Raskoff (1994) and Bradley (1995; 1997, as cited in Welch, 1999), focusing on three main aspects of reflection: (a) affect (what and how students felt), (b) behavior (what the students did and how students behaved before, during, and after the experience), and (c) cognition (what students learned). The ABC123s was informed by the work by Yates and Youniss (1996, 1997), adding the three points of awareness in reflection: (a) self, (b) other/empathetic, and (c) systematic/global (Dubinsky et al., 2012; Welch, 1999; Welch & James, 2007). Both models were organized into a template and rubrics by Welch (1999) for helping students understand what to consider during their reflection and for guiding faculty on what reflection needs to include (Welch & James, 2007). The intention of this reflection model is to promote both empowerment and responsibility in learners (Dubinsky et al., 2012). Learners are the only individuals who can process the meaning of their experiences and turn their experiences into learning. Both ABCs and ABC123s reflection models invite students to reflect holistically and from multiple perspectives. Unlike mathematical problems, there is no right answer that can confirm the meaning of the experience. Engaging students in this reflective process is not only for gaining insights but also for taking ownership of their learning.

By using the ABCs and ABC123s as a model for creating reflective narratives[1], we take students through a series of writing assignments that systematically build their reflective writing skills. Starting with getting students familiar with the genre and comfortable creating reflective writing, we build their skills through four years to the point where they can create stories that function as acts of transformational learning.

Year 1: Just Do It

Our first-year reflection assignments focus on establishing a baseline for students to pay attention, select their own topics of reflection, and use narrative to contain their experiences for further examination. Our goal, therefore, is to offer multiple opportunities for students to practice reflective writing and become comfortable reflecting on their experiences. We call this the "Just Do It" Approach.

In the process of designing reflective writing assignments, we considered that many first-year students have little to no experience reflecting on themselves, which may require them to integrate their personal thoughts, emotions, and behaviors in an academic setting. In his article on reflection in the student affairs field, Johnson (2009) points out that many students (especially those from the millennial generation) enter college with skills in collaborating and multitasking but do not have much practice reflecting on their own experiences (p. 87). In addition, Welch (1999) points to practitioners of written reflections failing to provide guidance on reflecting and argues that reflection must be taught. Therefore, the writing assignments designed for the first year were intentionally broad to allow students to write about a variety of different experiences and also included some specific guidelines in order for students to focus on specific perspectives or ideas.

One way we framed the need for developing more reflective skills among first-year students was to pose it as a necessary skill that helps incoming college students build relationships, enhance their own well-being, and succeed academically. In her article on reflective writing in first-year courses, Everett (2013) identifies several challenges first-year students face when transitioning to college, including "newly found independence, living with roommates, activities associated with daily living, homesickness and identity" and explains how many universities have created first-year seminar classes to assist students in this transition (p. 213). Everett studied weekly reflection writing from 110 students in four sections of a three-credit first-year seminar in order to better understand how reflective writing could be beneficial to first-year students both academically and personally (p. 214). Everett found that reflection writing was a useful tool for student health and wellness as it allowed students to "vent" or relieve stress about working through life challenges. She also found that reflection writing was a means of self-discovery and an important tool that allowed students to form a connection to the instructor, an important factor in students developing a sense of belonging in an academic setting (p. 219). Everett's research helped reinforce the Just Do It approach of quantity over quality as it allowed us to better understand the number of ways simple reflection could be beneficial to students.

TABLE 7.1 Perspectives, objectives, and example prompts for first-year reflective writing assignments

Perspective	Objective	Example prompts
Behavior	To describe a specific experience using specific, concrete details.	1. Describe a specific experience dealing with stress this semester. What, if anything, did you do to resolve this stressful situation? 2. Describe a specific experience working as part of a team. What role did you play in this team?
Affect	To describe feelings associated with specific experiences.	1. How did this stressful experience make you feel? 2. How did you feel about working in a team?
Cognition	To describe lessons learned from the experience and any connections to the larger world.	1. What have you learned about yourself and/or stress based on this experience? 2. How have these experiences working in teams impacted the way you think about collaboration?

The reflective writing assignments during year 1 were adapted from the ABCs of Reflection Writing and ABCs123 Reflective Writing models. Each assignment included a prompt that helped students view a specific experience from the three perspectives discussed in the ABCs of Reflective Writing. For the points of awareness discussed in the ABCs123 Reflective Writing model, students focused on the "self" and were not asked to reflect on the other/empathetic and systematic/global points. Table 7.1 presents the perspectives, objectives, and example prompts for first-year reflective writing assignments.

This framework allowed students to begin the process of reflecting on their experience and practicing the skills necessary in reflective writing. Many of the prompts asked students to choose a specific experience, often from the near-past, in order to better recall some of the specific details about that experience. Students practiced choosing which experiences to reflect upon and what details to include. Faculty assisted students through prompts asking specific questions that asked students to examine the experiences from different perspectives. While we didn't ask students to go very "deep" with their reflection or to focus on other levels of reflection aside from the "self," the reflective writing assignments in year 1 asked students to uncover new knowledge and meaning from their experiences – an important aspect of Nissan's assimilation learning style. This, we believe, helps students better understand what reflection could do for them personally and academically and helps us establish a baseline to build on for future reflection assignments.

Years 2 and 3: Deepening Exploration of Self and Others

Moving into the second and third years of UMR's health science curriculum, the practice of reflective writing continues and expands into many different courses. The goal of these years in terms of reflection is to help students intentionally deepen their reflections using the two different models cited earlier: ABCs of Reflection Writing and ABCs123 Reflective Writing model. Students are encouraged to think beyond their habitual perceptions and first reactions. The writing assignments move from a more self-centered contemplation to a more empathetic mode by becoming aware of the views of others and society. UMR's curriculum fosters this deeper reflective writing through a required series of professional development courses that all use the ABCs of Reflection Writing model in asking students to think about experiences such as job shadowing or volunteering and pushing students to go beyond a recitation of what they did and move into deeper analysis of their experiences, their community, and their world.

One specific course that is integral to UMR's reflective writing curriculum is a community-engaged learning course called Community CoLaboratory. The class includes multiple reflective writing assignments that build intentionally on the first-year reflective writing curriculum. The course assigns students to different community organizations with whom they complete a wide range of service projects and volunteering. They meet at least once a week with the community partner to complete their project and once a week as a class to gain the theoretical frameworks to help them make meaning out of their experiences. The three major writing assignments in the course are a series of critical reflection assignments that ask students to think about their experiences working with the community partner and critically analyze their experiences using course concepts. Unlike in the first-year reflection assignments, these critical reflections are assessed using a rubric that specifically asks for depth of reflection in all three areas of affect, behavior, and cognition. Students must now begin to really take responsibility for their own learning if they wish to be successful in the course.

The reflections themselves are designed with three-part prompts to invite reflection on the students' work in the community from multiple perspectives. The ABCs of Reflection Writing is explicitly written into the prompts through the use of three questions, one from each perspective. For example, the final critical reflection of the semester asks students to first describe a situation they experienced that illustrates their privilege or lack of privilege when working with the community partner. The first part of the prompt asks them to describe what happened (behavior). The second question of the prompt asks students how working on this project makes them feel at this point in the semester, which pushes students to evaluate their feelings (affect) about the experience. Finally, the prompt asks students to articulate what they have learned from the community engagement work and connect that to course concepts, encouraging students to make meaning out of the community experience using the academic material covered in the course (cognition). While the ABCs of Reflection Writing model is explicitly built into the course critical reflections, the ABCs123 Reflective Writing model is also implied in the reflection prompts. Thus, the prompts not only ask students to recount an experience and their feelings, but they are also asked to consider how others might feel, how their work may impact the communities they are working in, and how their work relates to larger sociological issues and forces. All of the prompts push students to move beyond reflection on the self and begin to think about others and the broader context using community and global perspectives.

Another set of courses that supports and expands on the first-year reflective writing skills are the communication courses available to BSHS students. Both courses offered are focused upon health communication, either in the context of patient-provider interactions or within the larger society, and both use reflective writing as a tool to help students connect their previous knowledge and experiences with the content covered in the course and to help them start incorporating social/external perspectives in their reflections. Like with the CoLaboratory course, the prompts for these assignments specifically ask students to include the components of the ABCs in their reflections, to include how others involved might have experienced the interaction, and to use course readings to help them make sense of the interaction. For example, in their reflection on intercultural communication, students are asked to reflect on a time when they had a challenge interacting with an individual from a different culture. They are told to include specific details about what they did in the interaction and how it made them feel. Additionally, they are asked to describe what the other individual did in the interaction and how they probably felt during it. Then they are asked to explain what they learned from the experience using specific course readings to help them make sense of the experience. This way they are using self-reflective practices to help them both assimilate new information and gain broader perspectives on their experiences.

End of Year 3: Greater Understanding of Self, Others, and Situations

The reflective writing takes on greater significance for UMR students at the end of their third year when they are asked to produce a proposal for their final year Capstone experience. UMR Capstone is unique. Unlike a typical capstone that involves conducting research or engaging in a special project, UMR Capstone requires all students to design the entire final year of their undergraduate curriculum. The creative and flexible nature of Capstone challenges students.

As the foundation for the challenging proposal writing, the first reflective writing assignment in the course asks students to begin the work of looking back on their time in college through a short reflective essay articulating how they have changed since their first semester. This essay is often a struggle for many students to write and complete. As most of our students want to pursue careers in health care, many of them do not see the usefulness of writing about themselves when what they want to do is help others. A small percentage of students are highly resistant to talking about themselves in a meaningful way, and they write about their growth only from a surface level with little detail, emotion, or self-reflection.

The second small reflective writing assignment for the course asks students to reflect on a conflict they have experienced while at UMR and think about what they learned about themselves and others. These two assignments show the same progression as the earlier curriculum with a move from the personal level to a more empathetic perspective. Students are also required to go through a peer review process for their essays that involves pulling up their essays on their computer, standing up, and sitting down at another student's computer. They go through this process twice and are asked to leave their table to review essays by students they may not know as well. This process makes many students feel exposed or vulnerable as they share personal stories and experiences, but it also reinforces the empathetic level of learning and makes them take their own reflection more seriously as they know they will be sharing it.

After these smaller reflective writing assignments, students begin work on their formal Capstone proposal. The first step of proposal writing is for students to determine what else they need to learn and how else they can grow. In this reflection, they develop three learning objectives that connect their past experiences to future career goals through their proposed activities. Simultaneously, they research and review a wide range of options for their potential Capstone activities. This process often overwhelms students. Previously, their academic experience was formed by simply selecting courses offered by the program. Now they are asked to design their own curriculum, and only they know if this design is right for them. Engaging in this process shifts their learning from mostly cognitive to deeply emotional. They are forced to break down their previous experiences to identify activities that they need. This evaluation process in itself is a reflection. Furthermore, they must weave all of this information together in a way that is professional and still personal. They must select particular experiences and stories to share to highlight where their goals and interests come from and demonstrate their readiness to take on this individualized learning plan. The proposal goes through a formal review process by an interdisciplinary faculty committee, and students must have an approved proposal to pass the course and begin their Capstone work.

While many students dive into the Capstone planning and proposal process enthusiastically, a small number of students offer a good deal of resistance to the reflective nature of the process. For some students, after two years of an intense science curriculum, they are just beginning to come to terms with changing career paths. Students changing direction after years of declaring themselves future physicians often struggle with the proposal writing course because they feel as if their lives are falling apart. Having to write about what other fields or work they might want to explore triggers deep anxiety and uncertainty. In some ways, these students are experiencing the type of learning Nissen (1970, as cited in Illeris, 2004) termed *accommodation*. They are being forced to break down their previous understanding of themselves, and this emotional learning can be difficult and painful. Even students who are not changing direction might resist learning through the course reflections. They are no longer being told what courses to take and what to learn from them, and this lack of direction and control brings discomfort.

Despite the small number of students who resist the reflective proposal writing process, the majority of students eventually see building their plans and writing their essays as a powerful tool for taking ownership of their education since they must construct a cohesive, individualized plan and convincingly connect their plan to their experiences and goals in writing. In many ways, this proposal moves their reflection into a more professional realm as they consider an audience of reviewers and make meaning out of their own skills and experiences in order to pursue diverse professional pathways.

Year 4: Become Visible Through Sharing

During the final semester or two, students are now implementing the plans they developed for their own Capstone in Year 3. As discussed in proposal writing, UMR Capstone is a unique opportunity for students to personalize their learning during the final year of their undergraduate curriculum. Up until now, students experienced cognitive, emotional, and social dimensions of learning within the framework of academic programs. The vast amount of time was spent in interacting with faculty and peers. University was the central location where the learning occurred. As a result, many students often identify a need to expand the social dimension of learning in their proposal. For example, many students include the navigation of ambiguity as one of their learning objectives and include an activity that takes them out of their comfort zone. The planning process allowed them to imagine their growth and become excited by their own plan, yet the reality of "doing" the plan provokes strong emotional reactions and demands students understand their situations differently. Thus, during the implementation phase, all Capstone students are engaged in the Capstone Reflections course.

This course is dedicated to one specific intention: engaging in the act of reflecting. At this stage of reflection, the aim is to engage students in all three levels of awareness, addressed in the ABC123 Model (self, other/empathetic, and systematic/political/culture). Students are challenged to hold more than one perspective and travel between multiple perspectives (Welch & James, 2007; Yates and Youniss, 1996, 1997). As the students navigated new experiences, relationships, and environments, both the ABC and ABC123 Models guide them to think from various angles. This reflection challenges students to "move" their stance. This course incorporates consistent communication and feedback, which are critical to well-designed reflection. Specifically, the course incorporates the following: (1) on-going implementation of reflective writing assignments and feedback from the Capstone Reflections course instructors throughout the semester, and (2) interaction with peers and the Capstone adviser, a faculty member who is assigned to each student to help them reflect on their learning outcomes. With this increased responsibility and complexity of their learning environment, being able to change their perspective is a crucial practice for students. The instructions during this stage strive to connect to the skill students need to gain before they graduate: the ability to handle, navigate, and process a wide range of unknown situations and challenges in the future (Illeris, 2004). This final stage of multiyear reflective practice pushes students to think flexibly and handle complex ways of viewing and thinking.

Reflection Writing Assignments

The reflection assignments are structured so that each requires students to critically analyze articles or videos that are likely to be meaningful and relevant, allowing students to apply them to their experience. The objective is to challenge students to have "a reflective thought," a conclusion that is derived from "active, persistent, and careful observation" of various pieces of evidence that exists in the beliefs students hold (Dewey, 1910, as cited in Dubinsky et al., 2012). Table 7.2, below, presents the list of themes and objectives assigned and their order. These topics were considered to be relevant to students' reflective practice at this stage.

Non-learning. The instructions for the Capstone course intend to provoke curiosity by asking students to respond to the topics listed above. However, in the process of reflection, students may need to process difficult thoughts and emotions. Some students may become overwhelmed. Others may have a defensive reaction. These reactions can turn into resistance to reflection. For example, the assignment on multiple perspectives requires students to admit that they held a single view and analyze why they did so by utilizing the ABC123 model. Some students express their embarrassment. Others claim that there was no other way to view their situation. In defining what is considered a successful reflection, it is important to acknowledge that resistance, too, is a part of the process. Learning requires students' openness to admit their own shortcomings. This critical evaluation is extremely difficult for some. As a result, some students may reject the practice of reflection and perceive reflective practice as unnecessary and uncomfortable. These students return to the cognitive dimension of learning as ultimately more valuable. As Illeris (2003, 2004) indicated, active resistance is critical for learning eventually, and educators of reflection writing must be aware that some learners will resist this practice. Reflection provokes a social dimension of learning, requiring students to reconstruct the way they learn. Educators must remain patient and be ready to provide a response that defuses students' defensiveness (Mezirow, 1981, 1985, 1990).

TABLE 7.2 Themes and objectives assigned and their order

Theme	Reflective practice objectives
1. Storytelling as an act of leadership	"Why stories matter" by a sociologist, Marshall Ganz (2009), claims that the art of leadership requires storytelling, consisting of three parts: the story of self, the story of us, and the story of now. Students are invited to first analyze why taking the authorship of their own experience and sharing their own story with others are valuable, according to Ganz. Then they are invited to think about the concept of storytelling as a form of leadership, how sharing about their Capstone experience can be an act of leadership.
	This activity aims to provide the larger framework of why they reflect and why the insights gained from reflection need to be shared. Students are specifically asked to identify the experience of facing uncertainty and how this story may inspire others.
2. Authenticity	How do we share the stories that feel true to us? Elizabeth Lesser's Ted Talk presentation (2016), "Say your truths and seek them in others," discusses the value of truthtelling and addresses our tendency to try to fit into society.
	This activity emphasizes the expression of their reflection. Students need to find a mode of communication that matches their learning from their reflective work. By using the ABC Model, they may come to a deeper understanding of their experience. Yet because they have not practiced communicating their new insights, they often try to fit their learning into the typical learning outcomes that already exist and are used by society at large. Through the concept of truth-telling as an important element to authenticity, students are challenged not only to reflect holistically but also to express their reflection accurately to their own experience.
3. Vulnerability	How does it feel to share our experiences, emotions, and insights? Vulnerable. "The power of vulnerability," by Brené Brown (2011), discusses how her research findings impacted her personally. She highlights the value of vulnerability by being vulnerable, including her own personal experience and emotions to support her main point.
	This activity aims to prepare students to share the final learning outcomes gained through their reflection. Sharing our reflection is a vulnerable experience. Students are instructed to identify some stories that they would like to share but feel vulnerable doing so. This writing assignment provides a safe environment to test and explore what stories need to be told and why.

(*Continued*)

TABLE 7.2 (Continued)

Theme	Reflective practice objectives
4. Multiple perspectives	What is the consequence of holding a single perspective? Chimamanda Adichie (2009) explains how holding only a single story leads to misunderstandings in her TedTalk presentation, "The danger of a single story."
	The aim of this activity is to emphasize that the inability to reflect holistically and hold multiple views leads to real consequences. The ABC123 model is relevant as students are asked to identify a perspective or understanding that they held before Capstone which was challenged during their Capstone experience. This activity encourages students to understand why their narrow view existed. Through this activity, they recognize how their self-view was constructed and also cracked by exposure to others and the larger society's point of view.
5. Navigating differences	How do we navigate differences to arrive at productive conversations instead of shaming, blaming, and fighting? Loretta J. Ross (2021), an activist and scholar, discusses how to build a culture that invites people to hold difficult conversations in her TedTalk presentation, "Don't call people out."
	The aim of this activity is to reflect on a specific situation when students remained silent or were called out and the situation ended badly or remained unresolved. Then students are asked to write how they might have handled the situation differently by using the calling-in, calling-on perspective introduced by Toss. This is an imagination and reflection-based exercise. The goal is not to solve the problem, but to identify effective approaches that are only realized retrospectively, with such approaches being useful in the future.
6. Critical incident	This assignment invites students to describe an incident that they considered to be significant because it challenged them to identify their own assumptions, evaluate their beliefs, and/or change their behaviors. The experience must have occurred during their Capstone. The students are asked to describe what happened (Hand), How they felt (Heart), and analyze why this incident is significant (Head.) In addition, they are asked to describe how they might do things differently because of the lesson from this experience.
	The purpose of this assignment is not only to ensure that students practice holistic reflection using the ABC reflection model, but also to challenge them to reflect on the behavioral change. The response to the last prompt could be that students do not do anything differently. But for those who have reconstructed their learning dimensions and behave

TABLE 7.2 (Continued)

Theme	Reflective practice objectives
	differently, this assignment allows students to critically reflect and become aware of their transformative learning.
	The Critical Incident technique was developed by Flanagan (1954, as cited in Rich & Parker, 1995), who conducted research for the United States Air Force, with the assumption that describing a critical incident reveals both effective and ineffective behaviors. Since then, this technique has been modified and used not only as a research tool, but also as an assignment for healthcare professionals (Rich & Parker, 1995).

Public Presentation

The final stage, a public presentation of the students' reflection to the campus and larger community, is an active component of reflective practice. The transition from written reflection to public presentation requires students to transform their learning into the act of sharing their insights with their community. As Fisher (1987) indicated in *Human communication as narration*, story-telling supports the process of meaning-making and functions as a mode of communication with others. During the preparation for this final stage, the students' framework of reflection expands. Telling their story of their learning outcomes and growth naturally requires them to reflect back to before they began their own Capstone. Suddenly, students face many relevant details from their past, some going as far back as childhood. Integrating everything into a concise and clear story in a real and meaningful manner becomes overwhelming.

With such pressure, appropriate support is needed. During preparation for the final presentation, students' interactions expand from communicating with the instructors of the reflection course to communicating with peers and Capstone advisers. They receive more feedback from various individuals, challenging them to think from a wide range of points of view. They search for the right language, visuals, analogies, and plots to articulate their experiences. By turning reflective practice from writing into an oral presentation, they begin to listen to how their reflection sounds. All of this deepens their reflection, which may provoke emotional reactions. Between the instructional team, Capstone adviser, and peers, as well as academic advisers, students are supported while learning is also facilitated. For some students, participation in this presentation itself feels like a crisis experience as they had never shared their personal stories in public. Students share their learning outcomes, which often include honest reflection on their failures, fears, and struggles that led first to self-doubt, then to a renewed sense of self and redefined the meaning of success. The nature of this presentation can challenge students to reconstruct their frame of reference, resulting in behavioral changes: transformative learning.

The final presentation has become a rite of passage, an important life transition, to demonstrate the students' readiness for life after college. This is a bold and unique requirement at UMR: every Health Science student presents their story and insights from their critical reflection publicly before they graduate. Such a condition is ideal for maximizing critical reflection. As Mezirow (1997) points out, our engagement in critical reflection deepens during communicative learning; the final presentation provides space for students to self-direct, critically reflect, and be creative to find authentic expression. The ultimate objective is for students to walk away from college with a solidified understanding of their growth and learning in college. This requirement to be physically present to share their learning increases accountability as students *become* reflective, health literate individuals. In addition, Capstone presentations provide the example to all students in earlier years that critical reflection is powerful and communicates the institutional expectation on reflection. This kind of practice has allowed our community to recognize the students' stories as quintessential in creating a culture of high standards. The students' courage to be vulnerable and share what it takes to learn and grow has shaped the practice and meaning of UMR Capstone.

Study on reflective practice during the COVID-19 pandemic

Thus far, reflective practice has been discussed as a tool for developing the mindset of future healthcare professionals. The reflective practice of gaining insight through awareness of the self, others, and environment was put into practice during the COVID-19 pandemic. Since reflective practice was already integrated into our curriculum, we studied how Capstone students used this space to process the pandemic's impact on their lives. Most Capstone students experienced cancellation of Capstone activities such as internships, research, and volunteer opportunities. In addition, students experienced numerous challenges including job loss, financial burdens, physical and mental illnesses, change of living arrangements, and the shift to online learning. We evaluated the meaningfulness of reflective practice through qualitative analysis.

Method

In Spring, 2020, Fall, 2021, and Spring, 2021, a total of 134 final essays were submitted by Capstone students. All students responded to the essay prompt, "What did you learn from your Capstone experience? How did you grow through navigating your Capstone experience?" with further instructions to include two or three learning outcomes with specific examples from their Capstone activities that explored the behavioral, affective, and cognitive elements of reflection. In assessing and extracting what is expressed from these essays, we used narrative inquiry for the qualitative analysis the codes that reflected common patterns in the transcripts were extracted; similar codes were assembled into categories. The narrative inquiry focuses on "inductive processes, contextualized knowledge, and human intention ... [It] is holistic in that it acknowledges the cognitive, affective, and motivational dimensions of meaning making" (Rossiter, 1999, p.78). Narrative inquiry also considers external and environmental influences, thus relevant and fitting in identifying the threads and themes regarding how the learning outcomes were presented in students' essays during the COVID-19 pandemic.

Results

From 134 essays, 323 learning outcomes were evaluated. The students writing the analyzed essays had the following demographic characteristics: ~75% female, ~45% BIPOC, ~45% First Generation, and ~15% transfers. Our analysis led to a final codebook composed of 32 codes nested within 6 categories. During the their Capstone, which was complicated by the COVID-19 pandemic, students reported that they synthesized academic content and current affairs (9% of total code frequency), became aware of well-being (16% of total code frequency), understood the purpose of reflection (15% of total code frequency), developed skills that strengthen relationships (26% of total code frequency), became humble and resilient (11% of total code frequency), and prepared for a future career in healthcare (23% of total code frequency). The table below shows the coding categories and their definitions. (Table 7.3) (Figure 7.1)

TABLE 7.3 The coding categories and their definitions we used for the essays that we analyzed

Category of code (n = 323)	Definition
Synthesized academic content and current affairs (9%)	Students reflected on their experience of learning course content that was particularly relevant to current affairs related to the pandemic and the violence against marginalized communities. Topics such as inequalities in the healthcare system, social determinants of health, LGBTQIA+ literature, disability narratives, and immunology were synthesized into students' daily and professional lives.
Became aware of well-being (16%)	Students reflected on what contributes to and compromises their own well-being. Such insights have been discussed as critical self-knowledge during the pandemic and for the future. Understanding their own needs also led to contemplating on what impacts others' well-being. This point was processed through their patient care experiences.
Understood the purpose of reflection (15%)	Students reflected on the reflective practice itself, why reflection is necessary during stressful times. Reflection is a pathway to becoming aware of core values, self-awareness, self-acceptance,

(Continued)

TABLE 7.3 (Continued)

Category of code (n = 323)	Definition
	what really matters to a self, and the appreciation of small things that often go unnoticed. Students also holistically evaluated, reflected on, and accepted a complex view of challenges during the COVID pandemic, encompassing the responsibility of the self and uncontrollable external influences.
Developed the skills that strengthen relationships (26%)	The art of building relationships is always complex. Students reflected on the importance of the following skills with a sense of urgency: intercultural competency, communication skills beyond barriers, the value of teamwork and collaboration, leadership skills, the practice of compassion and empathy, the rewards of serving, effective patient interaction, and advocacy, with the interest in building relationships and trust.
Became humble and resilient (11%)	Students reflected on their attitude and mindset as they adapted to constant changes during the COVID pandemic. Students reflected on showing up to difficult situations, taking risks by trying new activities that they normally would not do or be good at, and navigating vulnerability by sharing their thoughts on emotions with others.
Prepared for a future career in Healthcare (23%)	Students reflected themselves as competent applicants, gaining academic knowledge and research skills, and identified career pathways, which were the results of the Capstone experience.

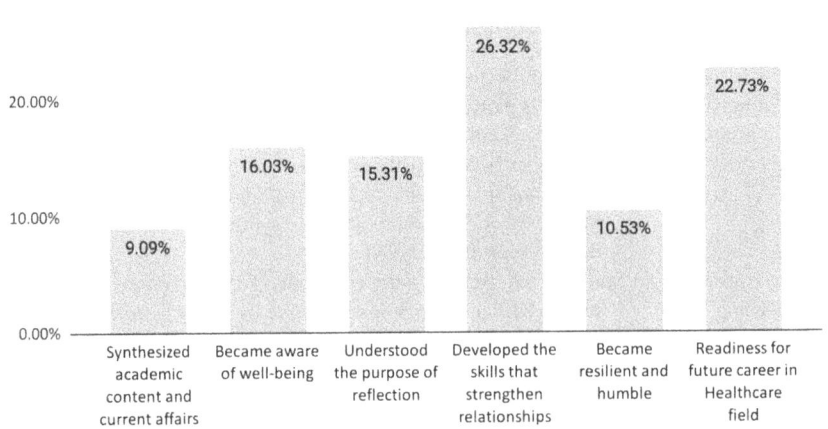

FIGURE 7.1 A bar graph showing the Capstone learning outcomes from the assignment sequence. Our analysis considered 323 learning outcomes from 134 student essays, and our final codebook included the six categories that you see here

Discussion

The results suggest that a crisis-like situation, such as the COVID-19 pandemic, influenced students to actually change out of necessity, reconnect with the self and others on a deeper level, and articulate the skills that they recognize as truly necessary for their future. For example, students synthesized academic content and current affairs simply because their current knowledge was not enough to navigate the COVID-19 pandemic. As students gathered the pieces needed to understand the instances of social injustice that they witnessed during 2020 and 2021, in the United States and globally, students connected the dots through reflecting on new information. Students often described these moments as "eye-opening," and this reaction contains mixed feelings of awe, from their eyes opening, and shock, as they learned their eyes were closed before. As indicated in transformative learning, this crisis-like situation pushed students to reconstruct their learning by opening up to new insights. These learning outcomes suggest that reflection during the COVID pandemic connected students not only to awareness of self, others, and the larger world conceptually, but many students also used all learning dimensions to change and become courageous, humble, and resilient. Making sense of an uncomfortable reality was only possible in such a situation. Making sense of the self in chaos is the heart of the pandemic narrative (Bird, 2022). Understanding of the self is not complete without understanding others, and students practiced all the levels of reflection throughout their time at UMR. The results indicate that the multi-year model of reflection allowed students to not only process challenges during the pandemic, but also to seek the meaning to find strength and focus. Such an ability to remain open and hopeful, while also dancing with the reality of challenges, is a critical skill for future healthcare professionals.

Conclusion and Takeaways

The sustainability of UMR's multi-year model of reflection is, first and foremost, based on collective understanding of reflection as essential for students' learning in the Health Science program. In what ways can we make the reflective practice sustainable beyond the classroom?

Second, the final presentation of UMR Capstone provides purpose to students' reflective work. It functions as the final act of reflective practice and also celebrates and reveals that students did not reflect alone. Creating an opportunity to showcase students' reflection could be deeply meaningful.

Third, the ownership of reflective practice must be beyond the instructional team. The construction of UMR Capstone, too, was a truly collaborative effort among faculty, administration staff, academic advisors, and the student engagement team. The instruction of reflection may be led by writing instructors, but the program and advice on reflection occur with various individuals. Thus, the ownership of this practice belongs to many, and the sharing of ownership allows the implementation of reflection beyond the classroom.

Finally, implementing intentional reflective practice means offering an ecosystem of support. Such support becomes especially necessary during a crisis. UMR had reflection as a community practice before the COVID pandemic, thus UMR's ecosystem provided the space for students to process their experiences, allowing them to share their reflection with the faculty and peers who were readily available. This intentional reflective practice supports the well-being of individuals and community, which is one of the fundamental components of health literacies.

Note

1 We chose narrative writing as our genre because of the familiarity of it, as humans most often process their experiences through the lens of storytelling (Allison, 1994), as well as use narrative as a way to derive lessons and meaning from those experiences (Fisher, 1987). Because of this, students can be more comfortable doing the in-depth exploration of their experiences that effective reflection requires, when provided the appropriate guidance on how to write an effective narrative. Additionally, narrative is a key genre in healthcare literacy, as narratives are used to provide case studies for students to analyze, are a key component of qualitative research on both patient and provider experiences, are an important means of changing health behavior, and an important tool for patients to express their symptoms to their care providers (Gray, 2009). Therefore, familiarity with the genre is useful to them beyond what they gain from their reflective practices.

References

Adichie, C. N. (2009). *The danger of a single story [Video file]*. https://www.ted.com/talks/chimamanda_ngozi_adichie_the_danger_of_a_single_story?language=en

Allison, J. M. (1994). Narrative and time: A phenomenological reconsideration. *Text and Performance Quarterly*, 14, 108–125.

Bird, J. (2022). *Reflections of writing narratives*. IGI Global. https://doi-org.ezp2.lib.umn.edu/10.4018/978-1-7998-9051-5.ch001

Bradley, J. (1995). A model for evaluating student learning in academically based service. In Troppe, M. (Ed.), *Connecting Cognition and Action: Evaluation of Student Performance in Service Learning Courses* (pp. 13–25). Denver, Colorado: Denver Education Commission of the States/Campus Compact.

Brown, B. (2011). The power of vulnerability [Video file]. https://www.youtube.com/watch?v=iCvmsMzlF7o&index=10&list=PL70DEC2B0568B5469

Dubinsky, J. M., Welch, M. J., & Wurr, A. (2012). Composing cognition: The role of written reflections in service-learning. In *Service-Learning and Writing: Paving the Way for Literacy(ies) through Community Engagement* (pp. 155–180). Brill.

Dewey, J. (1910). *How we think*. Boston, Massachusetts: D.C. Heath.

Everett, M. C. (2013). Reflective journal writing and the first-year experience. *International Journal of Teaching and Learning in Higher Education*, 25(2), 213–222.

Fisher, W. (1987). *Human communication as narration: Toward a philosophy of reason, value, and action*. Columbia: University of South Carolina Press.

Flanagan, J. (1954). The critical incident technique. *Psychological Bulletin*, 51, 327–358.

Ganz, M. (2009). Why stories matter: The art craft of social change (Organizing for Social Change). *Sojourners Magazine*, 38(3), 16.

Gray, J. (2009). The power of storytelling: Using narrative in the healthcare context. *Journal of Communication in Healthcare*, 2(3), 258–273.

Hondagneu-Sotelo, P., & Raskoff, S. (1994). Community service learning: Promises and problems. *Teaching Sociology*, 22(3), 248–254.

Illeris, K. (2002). *The three dimensions of learning*. Roskilde: Roskilde University Press.

Illeris, K. (2003). Adult education as experienced by the learners. *International Journal of Lifelong Education*, 22(1), 13–23.

Illeris, K. (2004). Transformative learning in the perspective of a comprehensive learning theory. *Journal of Transformative Education*, 2(2), 79–89. 10.1177/1541344 603262315

Johnson, J. (2009). Defining reflection in student affairs: A new culture of approach. *The Vermont Connection*, 30, 87–97. http://www.uvm.edu/~vtconn/v30/Johnson.pdf

Kerr, L. (2010). More than words: Applying the discipline of literary creative writing to the practice of reflective writing in health care education. *Journal of Medical Humanities*, 31, 295–301. doi 10.1007/s10912-010-9120-6

Koh, Y. H., Wong, M. L., & Lee, J. J. (2014). Medical students' reflective writing about a task-based learning experience on public health communication. *Medical Teacher*, 36, 121–129. Doi: 10.3109/0142159X.2013.849329

Lesser, E. (2016). *Say your truths and seek them in others [Video file]*. https://www.ted.com/ talks/elizabeth_lesser_say_your_truths_and_seek_them_in_others?utm_source=news- letter_daily&utm_campaign=daily&utm_medium=email&utm_content=button__ 2016-12-08

Locher, M. (2017). *Reflective writing in medical practice: A linguistic perspective* (Language at work; 2). Bristol; Blue Ridge Summit: Multilingual Matters.

Mezirow, J. (1981). A critical theory of adult learning and Education. *Adult Education*, 32(1), 3–24. 10.1177/074171368103200101

Mezirow, J. (1985). A critical theory of self-directed learning. *New Directions for Adult and Continuing Education*, 1985(25), 17–30.

Mezirow, J. (1990). *Fostering critical reflection in adulthood: A guide to transformative and emancipatory learning* (1st ed., Jossey-Bass higher education series). San Francisco: Jossey-Bass.

Mezirow, J. (1991). *Transformative dimensions of adult learning* (1st ed., Jossey-Bass higher and adult education series). San Francisco: Jossey-Bass.

Mezirow, J. (1992). Transformation theory: Critique and confusion. *Adult Education Quarterly*, 42(4), 250–252.

Mezirow, J. (1997). Transformative learning: Theory to practice. *New Directions for Adult and Continuing Education*, 74, 5–12.

Nissen, T. (1970). *Learning and pedagogy*. Copenhagen, Denmark: Munksgaard.

Rich, A., & Parker, D. L. (1995). Reflection and critical incident analysis: Ethical and moral implications of their use within nursing and midwifery education. *Journal of Advanced Nursing*, 22(6), 1050–1057.

Rossiter M. (1999). A narrative approach to development: Implications for adult educa- tion. *Adult Education Quarterly*, 50(1), 56–71. doi:10.1177/07417139922086911

Sandars, J. (2009). The use of reflection in medical education: AMEE Guide No. 44. *Medical Teacher*, 31(8), 685–695. doi:10.1080/01421590903050374

Sorensen K., Broucke S. V., Fullam J., Doyle G., Pelikan J., Slonska A., & Brand H. (2012). HLS-EU Consortium Health Literacy Project European. Health literacy and public health: A systematic review and integration of definitions and models. *BMC Public Health*, 12, 80. doi:10:1186/1471-2458-12-80

Wald, H. S., Anthony, D. A., Hutchinson, T., Liben, S., Smilovitch, M., & Donato, A. (2015). Professional identity formation in medical education for humanistic, resilient physicians: Pedagogic strategies for bridging theory to practice. *Academic Medicine*, 90(6), 753–760. doi: 10.1097/ACM.0000000000000725

Welch, M. (1999). The ABCs of reflection: A template for students and instructors to implement written reflection in service-learning. *NSEE Quarterly*, 25(2), 22–25.

Welch, M., & James, R. C. (2007). An investigation on the impact of a guided reflection technique in service-learning courses to prepare special educators. *Teacher Education and Special Education*, 30(4), 276–285.

Yates, M., & Youniss, J. (1996). Community service and political-moral identity in adolescents. *Journal of Research on Adolescence*, 6(3), 271–284.

Youniss, J., & Yates, M. (1997). *Community service and social responsibility in youth*. Chicago, IL.: University of Chicago Press.

8

WRITING ACROSS THE HEALTH LITERACIES CURRICULUM: THE BACHELOR OF HEALTHCARE STUDIES PROGRAM AT MUSC

Michael J. Madson, Elizabeth A. Brown, Elinor Borgert, Catherine VanderWerker, and Lauren Geller

In 2016, a new undergraduate program was launched at the Medical University of South Carolina (MUSC): the online Bachelor of Science in Healthcare Studies (HCS). The HCS program features a one and half-year online curriculum that prepares students for careers in the health professions and/or graduate studies. Many of the students in the HCS program are recent graduates of local community colleges, and many have struggled with academic and scientific writing. Yet, by the end of their studies, they have strengthened a rich variety of individual and organizational health literacies that culminate in a lengthy practicum paper.

In this chapter, we overview the HCS program, which follows what we call a "health literacies across the curriculum" (HLAC) approach. We argue that an integrative approach like this can help prepare undergraduates for the individual and organizational demands of careers in the healthcare industry, advocate for patients, and be more informed consumers of the healthcare system themselves. Such an approach supports longstanding, national calls to improve the health literacies, broadly conceived, of undergraduate students (Association of American Colleges and Universities, 2002; Institute of Medicine, 2004).

Below, we explain the HLAC approach, which blends principles of Writing Across the Curriculum (WAC) with principles of health literacies. Next, we provide a brief history of the HCS program along with a snapshot of our institutional context. Third, we explain the curriculum of the HCS program, emphasizing the literacy training that students receive. Fourth, we discuss some of the program outcomes suggesting its effectiveness. Fifth and finally, we conclude with recommendations for health literacy instructors and program developers.

DOI: 10.4324/9781003316770-11

Conceptual Framework

Like the health sciences program featured in Chapter 6, the HCS program applies principles of WAC, which rests on the well-founded belief that "language, learning, and teaching are inextricably linked" (Russell, 1992, p. 41). The WAC movement has roots in curricular developments that took place in or around the 1970s when scholars such as James Britton, Douglas Barnes, and Harold Rosen persuasively argued that writing instruction should not be limited to the English department alone. Rather, writing instruction should be integrated throughout students' programs of study (Russell, 1992). In the United States, some of the earliest WAC programs were established at Central College, Carlton College, Beaver College, and Michigan Technological University. These programs featured faculty seminars and workshops on the teaching of writing, writing intensive course requirements, and peer tutoring (Bazerman et al., 2005, p. 26), which remain common elements of WAC programs today.

A growing number of scholars have examined the application of WAC principles in health-related programs. In the 1980s and 1990s, the WAC movement attracted limited attention from scholars in allied health (Wesolowski, 1986), pharmacy (Hobson, 1996; Hobson & Lerner, 1999; see also Lerner, 2001), and nursing (Devlin & Slaninka, 1981; Lashley & Wittstadt, 1993; Slimmer, 1992). Since then, WAC has become increasingly popular in nursing education (Hawks et al., 2016), as WAC can help students not just improve their written communication skills, but acquire knowledge in challenging subjects such as pathophysiology (Hepburn et al., 2018). As Mackenzie (2018) explained, referring to public health education, "Integrating WAC changes how higher education is delivered, from a lecture-and-examination-based model to one that is more student-centered, interactive, and engaging (p. 616)."

In the HCS program, our HLAC approach incorporates principles of WAC. Writing is infused throughout the curriculum, and we calculated that students complete more than 50 writing assignments during the program, resulting in approximately 290 pages of work. (This total includes the practicum project, which typically is 70 pages long.) The writing assignments are a combination of "learning-to-communicate" and "communicating-to-learn," similar to the strategies that Thompson and Hendrix (2000) identified in veterinary training.

As the name suggests, HLAC also incorporates principles of health literacies, which align with the categories that Nutbeam (2008) described. One is functional, which comprises the basic reading and writing skills that students need for everyday situations. A second is interactive, referring to more advanced socio-cognitive skills cognitive, and social skills that allow students to extract and apply new information amid shifting circumstances. A third is critical, which enables students to critically analyze the information they encounter and gain greater control over their life situations. As Kasey Larson and colleagues discuss in

Chapter 2, critical health literacy is a valuable but often neglected set of competencies, including for students entering the health professions. To be sure, critical health literacy is needed today perhaps more than ever, and its foundations of critical thinking support the practice of evidence-based medicine, the demonstration of clinical reasoning, and ultimately the development of competent healthcare practitioners and critically literate health societies.

Along with writing, HLAC underscores the importance of reading – not just texts and data, but peoples and places. The HCS program subsequently has several objectives: Students will

- Develop an understanding of the determinants of health.
- Develop creative and innovative health interventions for diverse populations.
- Understand the strengths and limitations of research to interpret health data.
- Apply ethical and professional standards and values to health professions practice.

These objectives are intended to promote students' professional development, preparing them for careers in health promotion or for graduate education. Thus, students receive extensive exposure to interprofessional education, which fosters competencies such as reflection, shared decision making, and conflict resolution, along with understanding of team members' roles and knowledge of values and ethics (Spaulding et al., 2021).

Institutional History and Context

The HCS program is located at MUSC, an academic health sciences center located in the Southeastern United States. MUSC was founded in 1824, making it "home to the oldest medical school in the South as well as the state's only integrated academic health sciences center, with a unique charge to serve the state through education, research and patient care." Every year, MUSC trains more than 3,000 students and 850 residents and fellows across six colleges: Dental Medicine, Graduate Studies, Health Professions, Medicine, Nursing, and Pharmacy (MUSC, n.d.).

The HCS program belongs to the College of Health Professions, which offers additional degree programs at the masters and doctoral levels. Masters programs include cardiovascular perfusion, health administration, health informatics, physician assistant studies, and speech-language pathology. Doctoral programs include health administration, nurse anesthesia practice, occupational therapy, physical therapy, and health and rehabilitation science. Across programs, students have access to one of the first writing centers established specifically for the health professions. The writing center is staffed by tenure-track faculty members who hold doctoral degrees in literature, writing studies, rhetoric, and neuroscience, and who offer individual consultations for students as well as support for faculty (Ariail et al., 2013; Smith et al., 2011).

Beyond the college, the HCS program was designed to promote the social good, serving the people of South Carolina. The state has needed ways to make higher education more accessible, including financially. In 2013, three years before the HCS program was launched, South Carolina students had some of the highest average student loan debt for graduates of four-year institutions ($29,092 per graduate). Moreover, South Carolina has some of the highest rates of preventable illnesses in the country, and the state needs greater diversity in its healthcare workforce. As explained in the program proposal, "This is especially important in the healthcare field because a more diverse healthcare workforce improves health outcomes for diverse communities, which bear the burden of many of the state's poor health outcomes."

The founders of the HCS program consequently sought input from the state's system of technical colleges, where underrepresented minorities comprise a third of the student population. During exploratory research, the founders elicited comments from administrators at all 16 technical colleges, and all "expressed great interest in the program for their students and have emphasized the need for such a program for their graduates interested in health fields." In 2013–2014, a survey sent to technical college students showed that about two-fifths (41%, $n = 505$) "maybe" would be interested in applying to the HCS program, and about half (51%, $n = 629$) "definitely" would. Thus, it seemed clear that the program would meet significant needs of students, faculty, and academic institutions in South Carolina.

To enter the program, students must meet several requirements. They need to have completed 72 hours of college credit, including all general education requirements and a course in probability and, statistics, or the equivalent. While there is a preferred minimum cumulative GPA of at least 3.0 on a 4.0 scale, the HCS program utilizes a holistic admissions process. During this process, the admissions committee considers multiple aspects of a student's application, including when previous coursework was completed, improvements in grades over time, work history, demographics, and personal characteristics assessed through a personal statement, two professional references, and a resume. While it is not required, many students enter with an associate of science degree from a South Carolina technical college, and transfer partnerships have been established with Orangeburg-Calhoun Technical College and Spartanburg Community College. The majority (70%) of HCS students are underrepresented minorities, rural or first-generation non-traditional college students.

Thus far, nearly all students enrolled in the HCS program have been South Carolina residents. However, the program is open to students in any U.S. state, and MUSC has been approved to participate in the National Council for State Authorization Reciprocity Agreements.

Curriculum Overview

The curriculum for the HCS program follows a lockstep cohort model. Students take 49–50 credit hours that are spread over four semesters, lasting 1.5 years. This works out to 12–13 credit hours per semester, allowing students to attend the program full-time while also working full-time or part-time. (Most students do work while enrolled in the program.) Students complete their coursework online, and they attend two to three days of orientations at the beginning of each semester, in August, January, and May.

Year 1, Fall Semester

Student take four courses: Introduction to Health Behavior and Education (HCS 300), Foundations of Public Health (HCS 302), Social Determinants of Health (HCS 304), and Academic and Scientific Writing (HCS 307).

   Health Behavior and Education (HCS 300) introduces students to health promotion interventions, applying various theories and models. These include the transtheoretical model, social cognitive theory, health belief model, diffusion of innovation theory, theory of planned behavior, theory of reasoned action, self-determination theory, Bloom's taxonomy, pedagogy, and andragogy. Students also learn about motivational interviewing, social marketing, and additional strategies for planning interventions. Students complete four discussion posts. They also complete six journal article reviews. For each review, students read an assigned research article focused on health behavior intervention within a diverse population, then answer a series of content and evaluation questions presented in a two-to-three-page written assignment.

   Foundations of Public Health (HCS 302) focuses on the major disciplines of public health, including their history and development. The course examines public health challenges relevant to South Carolina, the United States, and the world, introducing students to sources of public health data, measures of health and illness (such as rates, incidence, and prevalence, and the role of law and government. In addition to online discussion posts, students complete a three- to four-page case study that cites at least five credible references.

   Social Determinants of Health (HSC 304) explores socioeconomic status, stress, social support, early life experiences, and other health factors, emphasizing health issues in South Carolina and/or the United States. Students learn theory and methods relevant to this disciplinary area, along with other current literature. In addition to online discussion posts, students complete a photograph essay and final reflection paper. The photograph essay prompts students to take a photograph in their local community, then discuss, over four to five pages, how the photograph illustrates a social determinant of health. Students are encouraged to avoid conflict, use discretion, and respect privacy.

The final reflection essay has two parts. First, students watch the documentary film *13th*, directed by Ava Duvernay, by the end of the semester. Second, they write a four to five-page paper that explores the various social determinants of health that the documentary illustrates.

Academic and Scientific Writing **(HCS 307),** taught by a writing specialist, takes students through five units that involve extensive reading on a chosen topic, discussion posts, and formal writing assignments. The first unit is learning to write, and students develop shareable guides on composition pedagogy, time management, and online learning.

The second is biomedical ethics, which culminates in a memo addressed to senior administrators at MUSC. Positioning students as communication specialists, the memo discusses what medical writing is, how prevalent it is, and what the university policies should be, in light of the four biomedical ethical principles (respect for autonomy, beneficence, non-maleficence, and justice).

The third is health literacy, which emphasizes not just textual communication, but visual communication. In this unit, students design health education materials in response to two scenarios described in Appendix A.

The fourth is qualitative interviews. Students identify a subject matter expert in their intended field, interview them, and write up what they learn in IMRaD format (introduction, methods, results, and discussion).

The fifth is teamwork and interprofessional education. Working in teams, students write position papers as hypothetical members of the Southern Group on Educational Affairs (SGEA), which extends from Virginia to Texas. The white papers address three questions: How should the SGEA define interprofessional education? What should it consist of? How should we promote it in the SGEA administrative region? The course concludes with a reflection on the five units.

A particularly important part of the course is the rewrite policy. Except for discussion posts, which are time sensitive, students can rewrite assignments for a higher grade. All they need to do is submit a new draft, along with a cover letter that explains what they changed and why. Students are not required to apply the instructor's feedback on their original drafts; they just need to provide some justification for their editorial decisions.

Year 1, Spring Semester

Students take Program Planning and Implementation (HCS 310), Overview of the U.S. Healthcare System (HCS 312), Etiology and Pathophysiology of Chronic Diseases (HCS 316), Principles of Epidemiology (HCS 324), and Practicum Development (HCS 330).

Program planning and implementation (HCS 310) teaches students techniques for clinical, workplace, and community settings. Students assess needs, develop measurable objectives, identify barriers, and employ visuals such as logic models and Gantt charts.

The writing assignments in this course are done in teams, and each is two to three pages long. The first group assignment has students conduct a community health needs assessment. In this assessment, students discuss relevant contextual information (such as county demographics, the health status of the community, the number and type of healthcare workers there), the specific problem that they intend to address, and a program plan.

The second team assignment asks students to develop a plan to address the problem that they identified in the previous assignment. Students consider the target population for the intervention, choose a theory to guide their work, identify community partners who might help, and set program goals.

The third team assignment prompts students to develop a budget and timeline, display them in a Gantt chart, and propose a program evaluation plan. These team assignments culminate in a team presentation, with slides, that students record over Zoom.

During the course, students can further develop their oral literacy by attending a workshop hosted by the university's office of Diversity, Equity, and Inclusion. The workshop centers on "having difficult conversations," which can help students decide on team member roles and set expectations for participation.

Overview of the U.S. Health Care System (HCS 312) explores the architecture of the U.S. healthcare system, including insurance plans. Students explain the dynamics of healthcare delivery, financing, and reimbursement; identify vulnerable populations, along with their health needs and challenges; and discuss current issues in healthcare reform. In addition to short responses on quizzes, students record an oral presentation that discusses the evolution of a healthcare profession. This presentation features at least 10 images accompanied by a detailed description.

For their final writing project, students write a four- to five-page book review on *The immortal life of Henrietta Lacks* by Rebecca Skloot. They consider characteristics of the U.S. healthcare system, ethics, public trust, and populations with special health needs.

Etiology and Pathophysiology of Chronic Diseases (HCS 316) starts with an introduction to foundational terms and concepts and a broad overview of basic disease processes. Students then learn about common chronic diseases that impact specific organ systems, including epidemiology, pathophysiology, and treatments, before discussing diseases that impact multiple organ systems. For their writing assignments, students complete about 14 case studies. As evidence-based practice is a pillar in the HCS program, students are also required to identify, cite, and discuss a peer-reviewed research article related to the cases. For the final assignment, students choose between writing an essay or completing an "un-essay" project on chronic disease. Both assignment options require students to describe the etiology and pathophysiology of the disease and support their ideas with scholarship. The professor encourages students to select a disease and/or project that can be utilized within their practicum, such as writing an etiology or pathophysiology chapter or developing illustrations. But this is not required.

Epidemiology (HCS 324) studies the distribution and determinants of health, disease, morbidity, and mortality across different populations. Students collect and assess quantitative data, learning about association and causality, the strengths and weaknesses of various research designs, and how outbreaks are investigated. Their writing assignments are primarily responses to questions that the instructor posts weekly, prompting students to think more critically about the course readings. Additionally, students complete a five-page report on a book with epidemiologic themes, such as *The fate of Rome: Climate, disease, and the end of an empire* by Kyle Harper, and *The chimp and the river: How AIDS emerged from an African forest* by David Quammen. They then read and comment on all their classmates' book reports, which creates a rich exchange of ideas.

Practicum development (HCS 330) leads students through formative activities for their practicum, a lengthy, final paper required for graduation. The practicum project is developed and written over one academic year. Typically, the final paper is required to be 60–70 pages, not including references or appendices. In the early years of the program, students needed to identify a target audience, assess their needs, deliver an education intervention, and evaluate the outcomes. During the 2021–2022 academic year, students wrote an integrative literature review that follows the phases described by Souza et al. (2010), which could lead to a journal article or a research presentation at an MUSC event. As most of our students come from the community college system, this type of writing and the extent of writing is new for them.

The process begins as students meet with the practicum professor to brainstorm possible topics for their paper (a timeline for the one-year project is provided in Appendix B). The practicum professor's goal is to help the student determine a topic that is most relevant to their professional goals, that will help them attain a great job after graduation or enhance their graduate school applications. To better understand potential topics, students conduct initial literature searches and read key articles that they find. It is common that students will pick a topic and change their minds, find that not enough research exists on a topic, or narrow down their topic as extensive research exists.

After they settle on a topic, students collect additional articles. Students are guided to develop an organizational system, including creating folders for each chapter, saving PDFs of journal articles in appropriate folders, and saving articles with titles that explain what is important about the articles, as this helps when students are trying to manage 50–75 references. Students are taught how to use reference manager software, like EndNote. As this process is continuous and adaptive, students complete literature searches, read articles, and make adjustments for the duration of the project. Frequent check-ins with the practicum professor give students time to discuss their progress, brainstorm ideas, share challenges, and work through strategies to overcome those challenges

The final assignment for the Spring practicum development class is a developed topic, along with a draft of a practicum plan. This plan includes an outline for each individual chapter including subtopics of each chapter as well as the citations for the articles that will be used to support each subtopic. In this way, the plan helps divide the paper into smaller, focused pieces that can be managed by the student, reducing the intimidation of writing such a large paper. The plan keeps students on track and focused, as it is very easy to get sidetracked and spend hours searching and reading articles that are tangential to their topic.

Year 1, Summer Semester

Students take Introduction to Applied Research and Statistics (HCS 314), Evaluation of Health Promotion (HCS 318), Health Policy (HCS 320), Leadership in the Health Professions (HCS 412), and Practicum Development (HCS 330).

Applied Research and Statistics (HCS 314) has five learning objectives: (1) to teach key features of different research methods, (2) to explain basic statistical terminology and concepts, (3) to review medical/scientific periodicals or journal articles that present statistical inferences, (4) to show how research is used to inform public health and healthcare practice, and (5) to enable students to formulate research questions/hypotheses on health-related topics.

To these ends, students do not just read about research; they write about it. Students compose a four-page essay on the state of scientific research based on assigned reading. Later, they select a topic to explore in greater detail and compile a literature review table with 8–10 relevant studies. (The instructor recommends that students explore their practicum topic in greater detail. She also encourages them to search for both experimental and observational study types.) From their table, students then summarize and synthesize relevant points of five articles that they chose, which results in a 10-page literature review.

Evaluation of Health Promotion (HSC 318) helps students understand program planning and assessment in various healthcare settings, ranging from local health departments to international nonprofits. Students study qualitative and quantitative evaluation, explore ethical issues in this area, and find ways to tailor methods to specific contexts.

As in other courses, students complete a series of weekly short-answer question sets based on the course readings. They also have assignments that involve entering, coding, and graphing survey data in Microsoft Excel. These skills allow them to develop a 10+ question survey on an area of research that interests them, such as their practicum topic. For their final data analysis and report (10+ pages long), students write up their class data set as a research paper, providing the appropriate descriptive statistics, statistical tests, and/or graphs for each variable along with clearly written descriptions and justifications.

Introduction to Health Policy (HCS 320) gives students a broad overview of the topic, drawing on news articles, peer-reviewed scholarship, and case studies. Students analyze how ideology impacts policy development, examine theoretical models related to policy development, describe the environmental influences on policy development, discuss future challenges confronting healthcare policy, and assess the adequacy of existing programs and policies.

Aside from online discussion posts that engage with the course readings, students complete two main writing assignments. The first is a four- to five-page policy brief that summarizes a health policy issue. This brief needs to include at least one visual aid, such as a figure, chart, or graph, and five references. The second is an eight- to 10-page health policy analysis, composed with decision makers in mind. Thus, the health policy analysis should weigh different policy options for the issue at hand. In the final draft, it should include visuals and at least 10 references.

Leadership in the Health Professions (HCS 412) covers a broad range of leadership topics, including strategic planning, grant development, team building, cultural competence, and conflict resolution. Students write two book reviews of four pages each: one for *Who moved my cheese* by Spencer Johnson (2015) and *Dare to lead by* Brené Brown (2018). They also interview a healthcare leader of their choosing as in HCS 307, and complete a question set based on the course textbook.

Year 2, Fall Semester

Students take Health and Disease Across the Lifespan (HC 322), Global Health (HCS 406), Rural Public Health (HCS 410), and Guided Practicum (HCS 480) or an elective.

Health and Disease across the Lifespan (HCS 322) highlights how lifespan approaches can enhance health promotion. The course considers a broad range of topics, especially protective and risk factors for health, disease, and quality of life, as well as the leading causes of disability and death at each stage of the lifespan in the United States. The writing assignments are low stakes, and students can choose between weekly annotations and reflections. Annotations are posted comments (three for the week) that spur discussions of the course materials and encourage active, engaged reading. Reflections are informal and often personal one-page summaries of the student's thoughts on the course material for that week. Whether they select weekly annotations or reflections, students need to cite one peer-reviewed source outside of the assigned course material. For their final projects, the students negotiate with the instructor their individual topic related to health and disease across two different life stages: one stage selected from prenatal to adolescent, and the second life stage from young adult to end of life. Students are to discuss or present their topic in light of peer-reviewed research, then offer a reflection. Final projects can be in the form of an essay or an "unessay."

Global Health (HCS 406) takes a comparative approach to geography, social class, race, gender, and other factors that impact health and illness. The course also considers cultural differences, including how various countries structure their healthcare systems. For their minor writing assignments, students summarize weekly readings and submit a response to the film *Sick around the world*. There are also two major writing assignments. The first asks students to compare healthcare systems in terms of quality, cost, and access; decide which one is best for someone like themselves; and argue why.

The second focuses on the COVID-19 global pandemic (though now with the option to focus on monkeypox or polio instead). Students are prompted to discuss six reasons why the world was more at risk for a pandemic than ever before, assessing the role each played in the pandemic. Then students describe six recent global initiatives that, according to sources they read, offer hope and (may) help(ed) combat the outbreak. While there is no page limit, the total length should be "at least 14 strong paragraphs." Students are required to have a writing center faculty member review an early draft and submit the feedback with their final draft.

Rural Public Health (HCS 410) examines challenges facing non-urban communities, such as specific diseases and disorders, practitioner shortfalls, and delays in service delivery. The course also covers promising community health approaches, rural healthcare ethics, and international perspectives. Beyond the discussion posts, students complete a windshield survey and a conceptual paper. The former (three to four pages) has students describe a rural community based on what they observed while driving through it. In their write-up, students may include a physical map and photos that capture community resources. Students are instructed not to go into unsafe areas, to respect privacy, and to practice additional preventive measures during COVID-19 outbreaks.

The latter follows up on the windshield survey. Students find a healthcare worker in the community that they describe, then conduct an interview on the worker's practices and perspectives.

Building on HCS 303, *Guided practicum (HCS 480)* helps students complete their written practicum project, which, at this point, requires 90 hours of work over 15 weeks. At the start of the semester, students meet with the practicum professor to ensure they are on track to write the paper over the coming months, and students start drafting.

Students are required to draft three chapters at a time, have the three chapters reviewed by the writing center, and submit them to the practicum professor for a draft grade and feedback. Each paper includes an introduction and conclusion chapter. Other common chapters include Social Determinants of Health, Research and Epidemiology, Pathophysiology, Health Policy, Rural Health, and Health Behavior. Additionally, students develop a questionnaire, generate data, complete simple t-test data analysis, provide interpretations, and discuss their findings and the implications of their findings. Students complete a reflection section that discusses their experiences and the lessons they have learned from completing the practicum project. The writing center reviews the final, cohesive paper and provides feedback to the student. The student incorporates the feedback and makes any final edits before handing in the paper to the practicum professor (see Appendix B).

Students are given the opportunity to determine a practicum topic based on their past experiences, future career aspirations, and personal and professional passions. It is very important that students thoroughly consider their topic and choose a topic they will enjoy researching and writing extensively about. Some examples of topics chosen by HCS students include "Health outcomes among transgender Black and Latinx adults and youth," "The effect of church-based health education interventions on type 2 diabetes among African Americans," "Best practices for dental health of autistic patients," "COVID-19 prevention: Utilization of the health belief model for face mask adherence," "The effect of COVID 19 on neurological outcomes," "Transaortic valve replacement (TAVR): Efficacy and safety for low- to high-risk patients."

As suggested above, the practicum sequence of courses, from HCS 330 to HCS 480, involves extensive collaboration with the writing center. The practicum professor meets each year with the director of the writing center to review the project and discuss progress and any challenges of the past year. They work together to develop a plan for the coming year, which is incorporated into the timeline provided to students. The director discusses the project with the writing center faculty to ensure that they are aware that HCS students are required to utilize their services during the coming year for an extensive writing assignment. Additionally, the MUSC research librarian assists students with their literature reviews and instructs them in the use of reference manager software to ensure proper citation management. This collaborative group effort and the strong support and mentorship provided to the HCS students have been pivotal in the success of the practicum.

In total, students accumulate 49 or 50 credit hours in the HCS program. Added to the 72 hours of prerequisites, the HCS program has 122 required hours by the time students graduate.

Program Outcomes

We collect and analyze several sources of data to track HCS program outcomes. Below, we summarize some of the findings relating to students' health literacies.

During the program, HCS students provided evaluations of their courses. Students who completed HCS 307, which spearheads the writing-intensive coursework, strongly agreed that the course improved their writing skills, confidence in writing, and appreciation of other healthcare professions – all important components of health literacies. Evaluations of the practicum courses highlight the benefit of staying organized, utilizing a drafting process, and giving students ample time to complete such an extensive writing project. One student suggested that "Giving us ample amount of time to complete each chapter, but giving us a time limit was very helpful and gave the push that was needed to complete everything in a timely manner." Another student shared that the practicum professor "taught strong organizational skills, which were instrumental in completing the senior practicum. The practicum required immense research about the topic of choice by the student. Without the info-managerial approach taught through this course, the senior practicum may have been highly disorganized."

HCS graduating students complete an exit interview and survey prior to graduation. Qualitative and quantitative data are collected. Qualitative feedback related to writing skills showed, among other things, that students particularly appreciated the support they received from the writing center. One student suggested that "The CAE writing staff members possess a highly admirable understanding of the English language. I regard them as impressive. I certainly hope these individuals receive kudos or the like for the skills they bring to the table." Another added, "I would like to thank (redacted faculty name), who was patient and took the time to review my work and guide me in a concise and effective way. I cannot overstate the challenges that come with drafting a review that is this comprehensive, and he was always available to help. One other suggested, "The CAE experience was excellent every single appointment and an invaluable resource throughout the program."

Additionally, HCS alumni complete an alumni survey annually. Of all HCS graduates, when asked how well the HCS program prepared them to "think analytically and logically" 100% of respondents ($n = 30$) said "well" or "very well." Similarly, when asked how well the HCS program prepared them to "write clearly and effectively" 100% of respondents said "well" or "very well."

After completing the writing-intensive HCS bachelor in science program, every HCS graduate who applied to a graduate program has been accepted. HCS graduates have been accepted into nationally recognized MUSC graduate degree programs including MUSC's masters programs in physician assistant studies, cardiovascular perfusion, healthcare administration, public health, and health informatics. Additionally, graduates of the HCS program have been accepted into highly competitive masters programs nationally including biomedical ethics at Ohio State University, medical lab sciences at George Washington University, health research at Washington University, healthcare leadership at Johns Hopkins University, and public health at Columbia University. Some students, extending their HCS coursework, have presented and published original research (Brown et al., 2020; Brown et al., 2021).

Alternatively, some students use their newly earned HCS bachelor's degree as a stepping stone to career growth immediately after graduation. HCS graduates have attained positions in multiple healthcare sectors including government (such as the United States Centers for Disease Control and Prevention and the South Carolina Department of Health and Environmental Control), in education as faculty and clinical program directors at community colleges, in healthcare leadership as program directors, in industry as clinical education specialists for pharmaceutical companies, and in nonprofit organizations. These are only a few examples of how students have successfully applied their health literacies.

Conclusion and Recommendations

We are intrigued and excited by the potentials of teaching HLAC, especially the successes of our students so far. Granted, the curriculum we share here is specific to our institutional context. Still, we believe that several recommendations can apply to readers' own institutions.

Infuse both high- and low-stakes assignments throughout the curriculum. Students enrolled in the HCS program complete a lengthy practicum project, which drives much of their final coursework. As we have suggested above, such a high-stakes assignment requires not just explicit instruction, but active mentorship to promote student success.

Leading up to the practicum, students complete a diversity of discussion posts, book reviews, article critiques, and other, smaller assignments that allow exploration in a variety of issues of health, wellness, and the delivery of care. The combination of high- and low-stakes assignments provides students with a broad foundation in functional, interactive, and critical health literacies (Nutbeam, 2008).

Support student writing through interdisciplinary collaboration. Most of the faculty in the HCS program arc health professions educators, and one is a writing specialist with a background in technical communication, user experience, and rhetoric. Yet, to ensure extensive feedback on students' writing assignments throughout the HCS program, collaboration with the university's writing center faculty has been key. Similar collaborations can (and should) be enacted at other institutions, though instructors should ensure that the writing center has adequate capacity for large assignments and staffing for regular consultations. Better still, programs could develop formal WAC programs that enact principles endorsed by the International Network of WAC Programs (see https://wac.colostate.edu/principles/).

Promote (visual) numeracy. Much health information is quantitative. As a result, we believe that instruction in health literacies must include not just reading and writing skills at the functional level. It should also include common statistical tests, the skills needed to critique various quantitative research designs, and some familiarity with data visualization. In our program, students gain this foundation in courses like HCS 314, HCS 318, and HCS 324.

Engage with policy. Much health information is also sensitive to broader contexts. Thus, we believe that instruction in health literacies should address regional, national, and public health policies, attending to social determinants of health. These may include the structure of insurance policies (as students learn about in HCS 312) or broad-brush comparisons between countries (as students cover in HCS 406), for example. Considering how entangled health literacies are in people's lived realities, we believe that instruction in health literacies cannot be divorced from discussions of ethics – a topic that we cover across HCS courses, and that Charles Woods and Noah Wason take further in Chapter 10.

Evaluate student health literacies experientially and performatively. Health literacies can be a challenge to conceptualize and, consequently, to evaluate. Yet, we have found that evaluations of student experiences and outcomes work well together, even in the absence of a fully elaborated model of what counts as health literacies. In the future, we hope to conduct additional evaluations, considering such factors as students' increases in self-efficacy and long-term development as professionals and consumers of health information.

In the coming years, we will continue to fine-tune the HCS program to meet the needs of our students. But given what we have observed so far, we are confident that the HLAC approach is a good one.

References

Ariail, J., Thomas, S., Smith, T., Kerr, L., Richards-Slaughter, S., & Shaw, D. (2013). The value of a writing center at a medical university. *Teaching and Learning in Medicine*, 25(2), 129–133.

Association of American Colleges and Universities. (2002). Greater expectations: A new vision for learning as a nation goes to college. Washington, DC. Available at: https://eric.ed.gov/?id=ED468787

Bazerman, C., Little, J., Bethel, L., Chavkin, T., Fouquette, D., & Garufis, J. (2005). *Reference guide to writing across the curriculum*. WAC Clearinghouse.

Brown, B. (2018). *Dare to lead: Brave work. Tough conversations. Whole hearts.* Random House.

Brown, E. A., White, B. M., & Gregory, A. (2021). Approaches to teaching social determinants of health to undergraduate health care students. *Journal of Allied Health*, 50(1), 31E–36E.

Brown, E., White, B. M., Helble, H., Gregory, A., & Geller, L. (2020). Identifying effective methods to teach social determinants of health. SoTL Commons Conference. 73. https://digitalcommons.georgiasouthern.edu/sotlcommons/SoTL/2020/73

Devlin, K., & Slaninka, S. C. (1981). Writing across the curriculum. *Journal of Nursing Education*, 20(2), 19–22.

Hawks, S. J., Turner, K. M., Derouin, A. L., Hueckel, R. M., Leonardelli, A. K., & Oermann, M. H. (2016). Writing across the curriculum: Strategies to improve the writing skills of nursing students. *Nursing Forum*, 51(4), 261–267.

Hobson, E. H. (1996). Writing across the pharmacy curriculum: An annotated bibliography. *Journal of Pharmacy Teaching*, 5(3), 37–54.

Hepburn, M. A., Myrick, K. A., Hakala, C. M., Pasquaretta, P. P., Foy, J. E., & Sanford, R. M. (2018). Writing across the curriculum: Educational strategies to enhance graduate/undergraduate nursing comprehension of pathophysiology. Paper presented at Nursing Education Research Conference 2018. Available at: https://sigma.nursingrepository.org

Hobson, E., & Lerner, N. (1999). Writing centers/WAC in pharmacy education: A changing prescription. In R. W. Barnett & J. S. Blumner (Eds.), *Writing centers and writing across the curriculum Programs: Building interdisciplinary partnerships*. Westport, CT: Greenwood Press.

Institute of Medicine. (2004). *Health literacy: A prescription to end confusion*. Available at: https://www.ncbi.nlm.nih.gov/books/NBK216035/

Johnson, S. (2015). *Who moved my cheese*. Random House.

Lashley, M., & Wittstadt, R. (1993). Writing across the curriculum: An integrated curricular approach to developing critical thinking through writing. *Journal of Nursing Education*, 32(9), 422–424.

Lerner, N. (2001). A history of WAC at a college of pharmacy. *Language and Learning Across the Disciplines*, 5(1), 6–19.

Mackenzie, S. L. (2018). Writing for public health: Strategies for teaching writing in a school or program of public health. *Public Health Reports*, 133(5), 614–618.

Medical University of South Carolina (MUSC). (n.d.). We're changing what's possible: The Medical University of South Carolina. https://web.musc.edu/ Accessed August 18, 2022.

Nutbeam, D. (2008). The evolving concept of health literacy. *Social Science & Medicine*, 67(12), 2072–2078.

Russell, D. R. (1992). American origins of writing-across-the-curriculum movement. In A. Herrington & C. Moran (Eds.), *Writing, teaching, and learning in the disciplines* (pp. 22–42). New York: MLA.

Slimmer, L. W. (1992). Effect of writing across the curriculum techniques on students' affective and cognitive learning about nursing research. *Journal of Nursing Education*, 31(2), 75–78.

Smith, T. G., Ariail, J., Richards-Slaughter, S., & Kerr, L. (2011). Teaching professional writing in an academic health sciences center: The writing center model at the Medical University of South Carolina. *Teaching and Learning in Medicine*, 23(3), 298–300.

Spaulding, E. M., Marvel, F. A., Jacob, E., Rahman, A., Hansen, B. R., Hanyok, L. A., ... & Han, H. R. (2021). Interprofessional education and collaboration among healthcare students and professionals: A systematic review and call for action. *Journal of Interprofessional Care*, 35(4), 612–621.

Souza, M. T. D., Silva, M. D. D., & Carvalho, R. D. (2010). Integrative review: what is it? How to do it? *Einstein (São Paulo)*, 8, 102–106.

Thompson, I., & Hendrix, C. M. (2000). Learning-to-communicate and communicating-to-learn in veterinary medicine: A survey of writing, speaking, and reading in veterinary medical curricula. *Journal of Technical Writing and Communication*, 30(2), 105–123.

Wesolowski, W. E. (1986). Writing across the curriculum in radiography and other college allied health programs. *Radiologic Technology*, 57(6), 534–537.

Appendix A: The case studies for the health literacy assignment in HCS 307

Design education materials in response to *two* of the scenarios below.

Healthcare administrator

Imagine that you are a healthcare administrator at a small outpatient clinic located in Gadsden, SC. After reading the latest reports from the Department of Health and Environmental Control (DHEC), you become concerned about the incidence of HIV/AIDS in your county—which is among the highest in the state. As a modest start, you decide to leverage the clinic's "health literacy environment": you decide to develop education materials on the basics of HIV prevention, which the clinic staff will review for accuracy and display in the clinic's waiting area. They remind you that many of the clinic patients, including young parents, are struggling readers who have only an eight-grade education.

OT

Imagine that you are an occupational therapist working in Saluda, SC, where a third of the town's 3,600 residents are native speakers of Spanish. You learn that the American Occupational Therapy Association is preparing for a National School Backpack Awareness Day, which is intended to help all community members—not just the students—learn how to choose, pack, lift, and carry their bags properly and thus avoid back pain throughout their lives. You decide to develop some educational materials that you can distribute to your culturally diverse clientele, some of whom understand little English, during therapy sessions.

Physician assistant

Imagine that you are a physician assistant who works in the Advanced Wound Care Center at Trident Health, located in Summerville, SC. An elderly patient who has a hearing disability presents with a chronic wound on her foot, a complication from diabetes. The doctor recommends negative-pressure wound therapy (NPWT), and although she consents to NPWT verbally, she later seems unsettled, saying that she does not understand what is going on. The patient is scheduled for a second round of NPWT during a follow-up visit, and to help her, you decide to prepare education materials that explain the procedure in some detail.

Perfusionist

Imagine that you are a cardiovascular perfusionist working here in Charleston. One day, administrators at the Charleston County School of the Arts send you an email, requesting your expertise. The deaf and hard of hearing classes there have been studying a unit on medical professionals, and the students became curious about how a heart-lung machine works. To support this academic unit, the administrators ask if you can create educational materials on the heart-lung machine that the sixth graders can easily understand.

Dentistry/Public health

Imagine that you are a dental professional who owns and operates a medium-sized clinic in Florence. According to the latest DHEC statistics, 52% of South Carolina children younger than eight have experienced tooth decay, and knowing your expertise in pediatric dentistry, city administrators ask you to design a billboard that raises awareness of this condition. They intend to post the billboard at the intersection of Highway 76 and Highway 52.

Physical Therapy

Imagine that you're a physical therapist working in Abbeville, where the poverty rate (nearly 40%) is the highest in South Carolina. At an upcoming town hall, you were invited to discuss how physical therapists can help combat the ongoing opioid crisis, which has hit rural communities hard. You decide to create a handout that illustrates your main points, recognizing that many of the residents have low levels of health literacy and literacy in general.

Upload your education materials to your group's forum for peer review.

Appendix B: Important events for one year student practicum projects

★Shaded boxes indicate the semester when the event occurs

Semester			
Spring	*Summer*	*Fall*	*Practicum Project Events*
			Expectations for Healthcare Studies practicum
			Spring course syllabus review (1 credit hour)
			Understanding integrative reviews
			Topic development/problem identification
			Research question/research goals
			One-on-one mentorship meeting with practicum professor, additional meetings as needed

(Continued)

Semester			
Spring	*Summer*	*Fall*	*Practicum Project Events*
			Literature search
			Research articles read
			Practicum plan progress report
			Practicum plan developed
			Summer course syllabus review (1 credit hour)
			Literature search continues
			Research articles read continues
			Literature review table drafted
			One-on-one mentorship meeting with practicum professor
			Practicum plan progress report
			Practicum plan completed
			Fall course syllabus review (3 credit hours)
			One-on-one mentorship meeting with practicum professor
			Six chapters drafted and submitted
			Feedback provided on writing and content from practicum professor
			One-on-one mentorship meeting with practicum professor, if needed
			Multiple consultations required with writing center during drafting
			Final review from writing center
			Submission of completed practicum

PART III
Extensions

9

CULTURAL HEALTH NAVIGATION AND HEALTH LITERACY SPONSORSHIP: IMPLICATIONS FOR THE UNDERGRADUATE WRITING CURRICULUM

Katherine E. Morelli

Having acknowledged the relationship between literacy and health, numerous researchers have attempted to define and operationalize health literacies within larger conversations about health equity, disparities, promotion, and access (de Leeuw, 2012; DeWalt et al., 2004; Edwards et al., 2015). As this collection can attest, health literacy (or health literacies) is a complex and contested term. Many definitions tend to focus on individual capacities. These definitions place a great deal of emphasis on the role of reading fluency and prior knowledge in understanding health and have been used and adopted by health organizations and government agencies alike. This includes The Affordable Care Act (ACA) that has made strong recommendations to integrate health literacies into the "law of the land," arguing that individuals with "low levels of health literacy are least equipped to benefit from the ACA, with potentially costly consequences for both those who pay for and deliver their care, as well as for themselves." Provisions include communicating health and health care in more "culturally and linguistically appropriate ways," and by extension, "readable" for those with low literacy levels. *How* to provide this kind of care is not always clear. One reason is that the role of language, communication, and culture in shaping, impeding, and/or fostering health literacies access and development has been under-theorized and under-researched (Sentell & Braun, 2012).

In this chapter, based on an IRB-approved research project involving a group of multilingual multicultural Cultural Health Navigators (CHNs) working at a refugee pediatric clinic in the southwest U.S., I present an expanded conceptualization of health literacies that account for critical factors like language, culture, communication, and even experience. Through specific examples of the CHNs work and their reflections, this chapter offers insight into the important

DOI: 10.4324/9781003316770-13

role that language, culture, and communication can play in terms of accessing and developing health literacies. The chapter concludes with a discussion of the pedagogical implications of these insights and offers recommendations and suggestions for undergraduate writing classrooms.

Background

CHNs are typically members of the communities they serve, acting as liaisons, links, and intermediaries between health services and their communities (American Public Health Association, 2009). CHNs offer a distinct category of non-clinical knowledge and skill sets based on life experience or "experience-based-expertise" (Gilkey et al., 2011). As multilingual "insiders" with deep understand of their communities, CHNs can facilitate important connections and relationships to/with the healthcare system and can be powerful "sponsors" for refugee families' access to health literacies in the health context. Sponsors of literacy are "agents, local or distant, concrete or abstract, who enable, support, teach, model, as well as regulate, suppress or withhold literacy" (Brandt, 1998, 2001, p. 166). After years of experience working within the healthcare system *as refugees themselves* and navigating the tensions between refugee experiences and medical culture, the CHNs became powerful sponsors of refugee families' access to and pursuit of health literacies in this context. Their experiences and the knowledge acquired over the years *as CHNs*, as this chapter shows, enable them to foster trusting relationships with families that facilitate greater engagement with the healthcare system.

Research Methods

To pursue this shared research agenda, I drew on ethnographic research methods (e.g., observations, interviews). Observations yielded nuanced accounts of the CHN's practices, tasks, activities, interactions, routines, and responsibilities. Interviews provided an opportunity for learning more about the views and beliefs of the CHNs, including how they understood the needs they were meeting and the challenges they experienced meeting those needs. Interviews also made some of the tacit experiential and intercultural knowledge that guides their practice more explicit. I invited the CHNs to reflect and elaborate on the insights and findings that were emerging from the study via a set of critical-incident interviews (Morelli & Warriner, 2021). The critical-incident-interview technique involves listening for moments where an account or story "got traction" or "raised tension" and helps to surface local "funds of knowledge" that directly inform decisions made or actions taken but are not always obvious or visible to others – even the CHNs at times (Clifton et al., 2016). In this chapter, I often use these incidents as examples and resources to think more about the role of language, culture, and communication in health literacy access and development.

Research Context

The refugee pediatric clinic, the site of the featured study, is housed in a comprehensive health center (formally the County Hospital), in a metropolitan city in the southwest U.S. The center treats both pediatric and adult patients and provides primary and specialist services. Most of the patients that seek care at this clinic are low-income and speak a language other than English. The refugee pediatric clinic offers specialized care for refugee and immigrant children with the assistance of a team of health professionals, including one attending physician, nurse, medical assistant, social worker, care coordinator, and five CHNs. The CHNs were from Burma, Somalia, Iraq, and Burundi. Between them, 10 languages were spoken in addition to English: Arabic, Burmese, Chin, French, Karen, Kinyarwanda, Kirundi, Maay Maay, Somali, and Swahili. Two of the CHNs were former refugees themselves and had spent considerable time living and working in refugee camps. Most of the CHNs had experienced disrupted education in their formative years, but all came to the position with college degrees and volunteer experience providing language support within their communities.

Working alongside the CHNs for a year was a tremendous learning experience. When we began the study in 2017, we were not entirely sure what we meant when we said "health literacy." Each of us had different ideas and thoughts, but eventually the countless observations and interactions as well as interviews started to inform our understanding of health literacies as well as the significant role that language, culture, communication, and *trust* play in accessing and developing health literacies. In the following section, with the CHNs reflections and testimonies, I identify some of the language, cultural, and communication dimensions of health literacy access and development. By doing so, the CHNs and I begin to develop a more dynamic, social, distributed, and collaborative understanding of health literacy access and development, which I expand upon later in the chapter. Building on the notion of "literacy sponsorship," we were also able to understand *why* and *how* the CHNs in particular are such powerful "sponsors" of health literacies for refugee families as well as advocates within this specific context. As Samira, the CHN from Somalia, once told me:

> I myself lived in a refugee camp from about 1992 until 2004. So, I know how life back home was in the refugee camp. How the appointment thing was never there and that it is first come first serve and how there often was no interpreter. It's hard to understand. So, now I know it's important that I'm here (July 12, 2017).

Language, Culture, and Health Literacies

According to the CHNs, one of the greatest barriers to care for refugee families was insurance. They often discussed how the concept of health insurance is new for most families they work with. This often means that the CHNs must figure out effective ways to support understanding without overwhelming families with information. This is usually accomplished incrementally with each visit to the clinic; the CHNs can respond to relevant and timely questions about health insurance that families need and/or want to know. In addition to helping families understand what health insurance *is* and *why* it is important, they also spend time working with families to fill out eligibility and application forms. The application process, as all the CHNs helped me to understand the demands of high levels of literacy in English, contextual and cultural knowledge and experience filling out forms.

In addition to facilitating access to services, one of the CHNs major responsibilities, is to make sure that families and patients have the "right" information. In much of the scholarship on language barriers in healthcare, providing interpreters and/or language support – whether in person or on the phone – is suggested as a critical "solution" to this potentially significant barrier to care and health literacies. However, as the CHNs helped me to understand, "sharing a language" does not guarantee accurate understanding for all patients and in all situations. For instance, Kriti once described a situation where she needed to clarify a patient's understanding of the meaning of the term "stone" in kidney stone (a term that was used in a diagnosis of a patient, but which had no direct translation):

> I have one patient it was from the hospital. So, the doctor said kidney stone, right? You have a kidney stone, we have to operate, to take it out, the kidney stone. So, the kidney stone, the way you translate is like we call in Burmese it's only one word … like *kyaut cut* right? So okay. But some patient, they speak Burmese too, but we have different ethnic groups, right? So, some different ethnic groups do not understand what *kyaut cut* is. So, o ok what is *kyaut cut*? What does it mean? So, and then she left from the hospital, and she said she couldn't sleep the whole night. The next morning, early morning, she calls me, "Kriti, why I never eat stone' and the body … if the body or digestion system it can make a stone in your body?" I said what kind of stone? I don't know. Yesterday I went because I had a hard time to pee and something and they check ultrasound and after everything they say I have a lot of stones in my stomach. Oh my god that's not right! That's not what they mention. Ok so do you understand what is *kyaut cut*? "No" – Oh okay, then now I got it. This is not the stone. You know the water sometimes when you boil water, right? Okay, sometimes you see the white under the boil. If you boil so many times and then it's stinky, white stinky, that's there on the pot. She said "Yes." Okay, exactly like this. You eat and then drink and the water is not clear, it can cause your kidney, kidney is a part of your body. So, I have to explain everything. (Kriti, September 8, 2017)

In this example, after Kriti understood what the woman thought was happening, she attempted to provide clarifying information. Observations and interviews made clear that this kind of "in-the-moment" interpretation was necessary but complicated and situated. For instance, when shifting from the families' languages to English, the CHN must imagine multiple potential contexts and audiences. In this example, Kriti needed to co-construct a way of talking about and describing what a kidney stone was in a way that was accessible and understandable to this specific patient. Knowledge of the patient's background was extremely valuable in this instance. Kriti knew that the boiling rice example would resonate with and make sense to this patient. This example also highlights how many languages are not all uniform and may include differences based on ethnicity, dialect/accent, or social and/or regional variation – linguistic knowledge that may be significant when working with interpreters and translated documents. As Reem, the CHN from Iraq explained in more detail:

> Yeah, sometimes, in some situations you cannot translate exactly what the patient says because, you know, it depends. As I am an interpreter for all the Arabic speakers so they are from different countries so … sometimes even them the patient, herself, she cannot give the exact word for about how she feels … that's why I'm looking for a word which fits that what she is feeling and what she is saying. (Reem, September 8th, 2017)

Testimonies such as these highlight some of the ways the CHNs shoulder the burden of figuring out the "right" way to communicate with refugee-background families in a clinical setting and the pressure that often came with this task.

The CHNs also discussed how they often had to help families understand the purpose of the medical encounter/interview and the kinds of questions that are asked. For instance, many refugee families were unclear as to why they were being asked questions about their medical histories. According to the CHNs, they often must help patients understand *why* medical histories are significant to the diagnostic process and *what* kind of information is needed. All of this (i.e., the clinical encounter) is new and unfamiliar for most of the families they worked with.

Casey, for instance, discussed how many parents struggle to understand their roles within the encounter and when (and if) they should speak and what they should say:

> The provider asks questions, and they're like, "No, you are the doctor, you know everything." But I remind them, he's the doctor, yes, he knows, but you help him to know about your kids. If you don't help him, he will not help your kid. Because you are the mom, you are the dad, you know your kid best than the doctor. It is you who guide the doctor to know your kid

and to help your kid. Because he's the doctor, if your baby has fever, cough, yes, he can do this, do this … but you are with the kid all day, you know how he is, you know everything about your kid. It is you who must … do not say, "You are the doctor you know everything." No, it's you, the parent.

Here we see how Casey works to manage the different expectations that parents bring to the visit (e.g., the doctor knows everything), while also helping the parents understand that *they* are crucial resources in the healthcare delivery of their children. When she says, "It is you who guide the doctor to know your kid" she is letting the parents know that the doctor needs their help and that they cannot diagnose and treat their child alone, even with their medical expertise. Over time and across contexts, CHNs scaffold parent-provider communication during consultations in ways that they hope will transfer to consultations when the CHNs cannot be present. This also includes encouraging parents to elaborate and expand upon any minimalistic responses such as just "yes" or "no" as this is common among the parents they work with at this clinic. These insights were extremely valuable for the attending physician who discussed the CHNs impact on the ways in which he communicates with families:

> I used to … I would ask the families like multiple questions at once. Like, 'Hey um have you had any fever, cough, vomiting, diarrhea?' So, Casey would interpret as I did … and the family would respond, 'Yes' and then I realized, Michael that's a terribly ineffective way of doing things you have to break it down and be more simple. And seeing how the families work with our CHNs I realized that I've had to most certainly adjust the way in which I communicate with our patients via the CHNs … that's definitely something that I've had to get used to and the cadence, the rhythm, the speed, the diction that I use is most certainly something I think I've adjusted throughout the course of this last year, and hopefully to the betterment of communication (Dr. Day, July 20, 2017)

The provider brings up a number of important points when communicating with refugee-background families at this clinic. Here he acknowledges it's not just what you say but also *how*.

In addition to developing (often on-the-spot) ways to talk about medical terms and concepts and navigate the complexities of accessing healthcare, the CHNs also commented on the importance of developing rhetorical skills needed to effectively inform and persuade parents and patients to take needed action. During an interview with Casey, she reflected on an incident involving a mother and two children from the Democratic Republic of Congo. One of the children had a hole in the heart and the other had tuberculosis. Both children were in need of urgent medical attention and care and the doctor and the CHN had tried on numerous occasions to communicate the urgency of the situation and the potential consequences of their inaction. However, despite the efforts to get the mother to come to the clinic, she never came. During an interview, Casey went on to share her feelings of frustration and concern during this situation and the critical role she played in raising the family's awareness of the children's serious medical conditions and the consequences of inaction:

> Every time I explain to her this situation, they need to see the child, if you don't do this with this condition, you will see one day, they can come to take your kid. And don't think it's me or it's the doctor because the doctor must report everything, because this is the situation where they must act and now … you can't wait. If they think the baby has TB, they must protect other kids. If she goes to school, they must protect others at school. If your baby doesn't grow right because of the hole in the heart, they must close that. You need to understand that if this is not … we are not here to play. We are helping you, and if we do not help you, I don't think you will get somewhere that can do everything how we are doing. (Casey, September 8th, 2017).

In this instance, Casey shared her concern that the mother did not know much about mandated reporting and other bureaucratic protocols of seeking care at a clinic (e.g., they can lose the opportunity to seek care there). Nor did it seem that the mother was aware that the child would not be allowed to attend school with TB. This kind of information is particularly important to refugee background individuals whose experiences have been marred by forced separation and disrupted education (if any education) – knowledge that was a big motivator for Casey and the other CHNs who worked so hard to keep families healthy *and* together.

The CHNs also do a great deal of advocacy work for their patients (in many ways most of their work is advocacy-based). This kind of work also played an enormous role in their capacity to help families develop needed health literacies while establishing more trusting relationships with the healthcare system. Over the course of the year, I heard a lot of troubling stories that required that the CHNs "step in" on behalf of the family. During one of our interviews, Samira, the CHN from Somali told me the following story:

> There was a situation where one of the providers. The patient came in and then she called me for interpretation. And then the provider be like, 'Oh um, why don't you speak English? You're in America. You're supposed to learn English since you go to Walmart and do your own thing' or 'Next time come in with your own interpreter, we don't have time.' Things like that I have to go in and tell them like … the rules (August 2nd, 2017).

When I asked Samira what she meant by "the rules," she said that she did not believe her patient was being treated fairly or with respect. She felt that the line of questioning and assumptions made by this provider were inappropriate. In this case, she called on a supervisor to speak with the provider. Samira added, "It's just you have to be there and show them, okay, this is not how you talk to this person and just make things clear between the provider and the patient so that the patient doesn't get offended, and the provider don't get offended" (August 15, 2017). Making sure that no one is "offended" and that refugee families are being treated with respect is such a big part of their roles as CHNs. Their ability to identify situations where families are being treated unfairly or with bias/discrimination (which is common) is yet another reason they are such powerful sponsors of the refugee families' health literacy development.

During the year that I worked alongside the CHNs, they also talked a lot about some of the challenges they experience in their roles and in trying to support refugee families' access to and development of health literacies. Collectively, we tried to understand some of the impediments to accessing and developing health literacies among their patients. One of the biggest impediments to refugee families' health literacy access and development was that the CHNs rarely, if ever, had enough time to provide the kind of patient education that they wanted to and that families often needed. As Angela, the CHN from Burundi explained, "Explaining the why and how is really a good way to give energy to the refugee families to start to do things better. To start to do things by themselves. We don't have time, but we need it" (September 13, 2017). The lack of patient education time was especially problematic when it came to medication and prescriptions since most parents did not read or write in any language. To make medication instructions more accessible, the CHNs often tried color-coding prescriptions to at least help families differentiate between medications. However, as Reem, the CHN from Iraq, put it, "We need more support. Sometimes we are asked to be two places at once. It is impossible to educate parents and families in the ways they need" (September 13, 2017). We all acknowledged that this was a problem and barrier in the way of families developing needed health literacies.

Unfortunately, without accessible resources to supplement what takes place at the clinic (and outside), so much is left to the CHNs to teach, answer, and respond to. If the idea is to open more space for teaching and learning opportunities while working towards families' greater independence, having other kinds of resources to support more independent learning would be helpful and could potentially open more space for teaching and learning while at the clinic.

When the CHNs had time, they did try to work on creating resources that could help facilitate interactions without them, but they had a great deal of difficulty in this case partly because they had no training or support in doing this work and partly because they weren't sure *what* to create and *how* it might be used by families.

Discussion

This study supports the idea that the CHNs are especially effective health literacy sponsors and/or mediators. One particularly significant reason is that the CHNs not only share a language with their families, but they also share cultural backgrounds and experiences (e.g., in refugee camps). As the CHNs testimonies show, sharing a language and cultural background were critical resources in terms of making important connections between refugee families and the healthcare system. Having more patient navigators and advocates like the CHNs making connections between underserved communities and the healthcare system is clearly needed and valuable. However, as the CHNs also helped me to understand, they were not well supported within this system and shouldered a great deal of responsibility. This is to say that while literacy sponsorship is an effective concept – it is only effective as long as there is a collaborative effort to support the sponsorship and the "burden" so to speak is on everyone.

The many testimonies in this chapter also demonstrate how locally specific and context-dependent the path to care is and what health literacies or being health literate means. Take for instance the "graduation list" the CHNs put together and shared with me when I asked about what they meant by "greater independence" as a goal of theirs for the families they work with. By "graduation list" the CHNs mean a set of tasks and skills they believe families need to be able to do to "graduate" from the refugee clinic and/or to be "health literate" enough in this context to do more alone. To health professionals that work in other contexts and with other patients, this list may not make sense or have value to them or their patient populations. They may wonder why providing the first and last name (or child's name) and date of birth would need to be listed as a "skill" required on the path to care. The fact that the skills are listed, however, is among the many reasons the CHNs are the most powerful and effective sponsors of health literacies for refugee families. They know, for instance, that many families do not make distinctions between first and last names and may not be familiar with the expectations and conventions of healthcare interactions. This is significant cultural knowledge that is needed to work with this specific population.

The CHNs work and support also highlight how health literacies are socially and interactionally mediated. Whether refugee-background or not, people rarely make health-related decisions alone. The CHNs often talked about how fast word spreads among their communities and how experiences with the healthcare system are shared. Testimonies such as Kriti's "kidney stone" incident also highlight the ongoing work they do with families to co-construct and negotiate new ways of talking about health and illness where there are no direct translations. Through this labor-intensive work, they continue developing their own intercultural health literacies in multiple languages making them even more effective. All this interactional support is critical in terms of trust-building between parents and providers. The more trust families have, the more likely they are to participate in the healthcare system and stay connected to it. All this work is situational, complex, and requires a great deal of time and effort – things the CHNs do not always have, especially considering the lack of resources for refugee families – whether human or material. Without other resources to support and distribute the development of health literacies in this context, refugee families continue to rely on the CHNs in ways that are unsustainable.

Interventions in Undergraduate Writing Courses

Undergraduate writing courses can play an important role in developing needed health literacies to better support patient advocates like the CHNs and more effectively meet the diverse needs of linguistic and ethnic/racial minority communities. In this section, I discuss several ways we can work towards these critical goals.

Language, Culture, and Health Literacies

Whether they enter the health professions or not, students must be able to navigate difference(s) and find ways to communicate effectively and appropriately. Knowledge of the cultural, linguistic, and communication dimensions of health literacies can support more effective intercultural communication and understandings in healthcare settings. Writing courses can provide the needed support in developing critical knowledge about the role of language, culture, and communication in health literacies. This can be accomplished in a variety of ways. One way is by utilizing reading opportunities in class to better understand these relationships. For instance, one assignment I commonly incorporate in my Writing in the Health Professions courses is a scholarly piece of writing. This could be a literature review, for instance, as this is a common genre within the health professions. To get comfortable with the genre and gain a greater appreciation for the role of language and culture in health literacies, we read about cross-cultural perspectives on health and illness; health disparities and access issues involving language and culture; different perspectives on the concept of health literacies and literacy more broadly from a variety of fields including literacy studies, applied linguistics, anthropology, and health communication. Readings support important dialogue about *how* language, culture, and communication can impact health literacy access and development across settings.

I also encourage students to draw on their own linguistic resources in their writing for class. Instead of viewing additional languages as a deficit, we reframe how we talk about language. We talk about language as a resource – a resource that plays a powerful role in health literacy development and in access to healthcare services. Students are encouraged to practice creating and translating documents created for class (or community partners) into language(s) in which they are also literate. In this way, they can continue to develop health literacies in multiple languages and/or dialects. Recall how Kriti needed to determine a new way to describe a kidney stone since this term or concept did not exist in their primary language. Often, students need to do the same in class when translating documents. They are not always able to have conversations with their audience like Kriti did, but the experience still highlights how meaning is socially mediated and negotiated through interactions and not all beliefs and ideas cross-cultural contexts.

Rhetorical Knowledge and Literacies

No matter what their career paths are, it is important for students to be able to adapt and *be* more responsive as writers and communicators. One of the key goals of undergraduate writing instruction is for students to become more flexible and ethical writers that *can* adapt to new and different situations as well as diverse audiences, which other chapters in the collection have emphasized. While we cannot prepare students for every situation they may face, we can provide them with rhetorical tools to help them effectively navigate the different situations and interactions they may encounter as they navigate the complexities of the healthcare system and the differences within it. Training students to be able to identify and analyze the rhetorical situation (i.e., audience, purpose, setting, exigency, context) and to draw on effective and responsive rhetorical tools (e.g., pathos, logos, ethos, pathos) are critical in supporting more dynamic communication. Rhetorical knowledge can also help support more critical readership of scientific and medical information, which is important for health professionals, patients, and caregivers alike. In the classroom, students can practice rhetorically analyzing health-related documents. These documents could be for patients, providers, researchers, and/or the greater public. Students can also rhetorically analyze a professional experience and/or interaction to inform future communication in that setting.

Usability and Technology

Health communication today comes in a multitude of forms and is written across a variety of contexts. We are increasingly relying on technology as we shift to more electronic and/or digital communication (e.g., social media, patient portals, electronic medical records); and while written English remains the dominant form (and language) of most health communication, we are seeing a gradual shift to more visual communication as well. All of this has further complicated the already complex health communication landscape and has raised important questions in considerations about not only *what* we communicate, but also *how, where,* and *when* we communicate. These are critical access questions and Charles Woods and Noah Wason pick them up in the next chapter. Recall in my study for instance, how health insurance information, eligibility forms, and applications were only accessible online by visiting the website or by physically going to the site. Neither of these options was accessible or possible for most of the refugee families at the pediatric clinic; and even if, somehow, they were able to access this information or forms, they still would not be able to *comprehend or use it*. For linguistic minorities like refugee families, this might present an impossible obstacle to accessing care if not for the ongoing support of health professionals like the CHNs. This is to say that in addition to analyzing the rhetorical situation, students should also identify and analyze contexts of use.

Contexts of use include factors like time (or the historical moment like COVID-19), geography, and environment. Once a health document (or computer program) has been developed, it is important that we engage in additional analysis: usability testing. It can be useful to consult usability texts in the classroom to inform student practices. A crucial aspect of usability testing is to determine where and how your message or project will be used, as Kirk St. Amant discusses in Chapter 11. In the classroom setting, this typically involves think-aloud protocols in which users voice all their thoughts (with some prompting from the tester) about how they are interacting with the document and what they are thinking, feeling, wondering, and/or confused by. Insights gained from this experience can inform the writer's judgment in making needed revisions to best meet the target audience's needs. Usability testing is a great way to get students to think more carefully about contexts of use as well as design. Seemingly, small decisions like font choice can make a big difference when it comes to readability and usability. In terms of thinking about usability, my students also tend to benefit by learning basic design principles and then practicing employing them in a low-stakes workshop setting.

Experiential and Service Learning

As Michael J. Klein illustrated in Chapter 5, the value of all skills and literacies students begin to develop and/or become more aware of is really brought home in significant ways when working in real-world settings through experiential and service learning. These experiences afford students the opportunity to work with real audiences, people, and organizations in the local community who *need* and/or *rely upon* the documents they create. Students also get the chance to organically establish relationships with community partners so that they can produce the highest quality work in a collaborative way. In terms of approach, there are a variety of models for service learning. The course could fully incorporate and center around the service-learning component; or as is often the case in my classes, students work on several smaller projects for the organization in groups or independently so that they have choices. Klein's students worked with Healthy Families and the Central Shenandoah Health District Center. The most recent organization I worked with was Asian Women for Health based out of Boston, U.S. This non-profit organization is a peer-led community-based network dedicated to advancing Asian women's health and wellness through education, advocacy, and support. Every student had at least one semester-long project they worked on for the organization. For instance, one writing project was to create an informational resource for Asian-American parents in the local area to encourage them to get their children vaccinated against the COVID-19 virus. The director's request was that the document(s) be across social media platforms and be accessible in physical spaces such as schools, faith-based organizations, or local clinics.

To pursue this project, the students and I met with the director of the organization to learn more about the target population and the goals of the resource and where she wanted it to be accessible. We began an in-depth rhetorical and audience analysis to determine the best course of action; this involved making careful choices about what to include, how to include it, where and when. Most of the director's questions about the resources we created had to do with use. Recall that this is something that students tend to struggle with and is one reason that service learning can be especially valuable; students get the opportunity to engage in the full process of invention, creation, planning, writing, designing, and revision with real audiences and purposes. They also are encouraged to consider decisions more carefully about context, usability, technology, and access. Sometimes students get the chance to do usability tests on live audiences, which is such a valuable experience. Live tests help students identify potential barriers to access and use. All this work – connecting to creating with/for organization – takes time, patience, and determination, but it is worth it as students stand to benefit from working and writing with real people and organizations who *need* or *rely upon* the documents they create.

Conclusion

This chapter reinforces the idea that health literacies may not be some "thing" that can be formally taught and tested in decontextualized settings. As the CHNs demonstrate through their work, so much is learned *in the doing* and as needed on *a* path to care, which is rarely an individual endeavor. For this reason, all the scaffolding the CHNs do and the guidance they provide for families in this context as events and interactions unfold is so important and useful. Based on more sociocultural theories of learning, the more families can learn in the contexts in which information is relevant or where practices and interactions take place, the more effective it is likely to be in the long run. With that said, it would be beneficial for there to be more in-context teaching and learning opportunities that account for and respond to refugee families' needs (e.g., language support) and limitations (e.g., transportation). This experience, the CHNs argued, was often missing, but crucial in terms of health literacy development. I would argue that this kind of learning is better suited for the situated nature of health literacies and how no path to care is linear, but rather, dynamic, and full of new experiences, interactions, places, and people.

During my time with the CHNs, I really started to see in very tangible and concrete ways how at the end of the day, health literacies are no one person or entity's responsibility. In a sense, it is all our responsibility. It is the responsibility of educators, health professionals, administrators, staff, patients, and local communities. In an ideal world, we would be committed to each other and each other's health and well-being. Unfortunately, ideal worlds are just that – ideal. In the real world, the CHNs continue to struggle to meet the needs of a rising patient population with limited if any support from beyond the clinic (and even within the clinic). We all acknowledged that this is not a sustainable solution to the problem of "low" health literacy levels among refugee families in the local community. Without support from beyond the clinic – in communities, schools, health organizations – the burden will continue to disproportionately fall upon the CHNs (and professionals like them) to keep refugee families and other linguistic and racial/ethnic minorities connected to and cared for by our healthcare system. Working towards more sustainable and collaborative efforts to understand and improve health literacies should be a goal of ours as educators. Writing instruction can play an important role in developing critical health literacies that can make this goal so challenging while identifying potential remedies.

References

American Public Health Association, Community Health Workers Section. (2009). Retrieved November 2, 2017, from https://www.apha.org/apha-communities/member-sections/community-health-workers

Brandt, D. (1998). Sponsors of literacy. *College Composition and Communication*, 49(2), 165–185.

Brandt, D. (2001). *Literacy in American lives*. Cambridge: Cambridge University Press.

Clifton, J., Long, E., & Roen, D. (2016). Constructions of critical incidents. http://ccdigitalpress.org/stories/chapters/roenlongclifton/ways.htm

de Leeuw, E. (2012). The political ecosystem of health literacies [Editorial]. *Health Promotion International*, 27(1), 1–4

DeWalt, D. A., Berkman, N. D., Sheridan, S., Lohr, K. N., & Pignone, M. P. (2004). Literacy and health outcomes. *Journal of General Internal Medicine*, 19(12), 1228–1239.

Edwards, M., Wood, F., Davies, M., & Edwards, A. (2015). 'Distributed health literacy': Longitudinal qualitative analysis of the roles of health literacy mediators and social networks of people living with a long-term health condition. *Health Expectations*, 18(5), 1180–1193.

Gilkey, M. E., Rush, C. H., & Garcia, C. (2011). Professionalization and the experience-based expert: Strengthening partnerships between health educators and community health workers. *Health Promotion Practice*, 12(2), 178–182.

Morelli, K. E., & Warriner, D. S. (2021). "It Depends Case by Case": Understanding how the practices of cultural health navigators impact healthcare access and delivery for refugee-background families. In D.S. Warriner & E.R. Miller (Eds.), *Extending applied linguistics for social impact: Cross-disciplinary collaborations in diverse spaces of public inquiry* (pp. 149–170). Bloomsbury Academic.

Sentell, T., & Braun, K. L. (2012). Low health literacy limited English proficiency, and health status in Asians, Latinos, and other racial/ethnic groups in California. *Journal of Health Communication*, 17(sup3), 82–99.

10

MAKING WELL-INFORMED DECISIONS: DATA COLLECTION, HEALTH INFORMATION, AND UNDERGRADUATE WRITING INSTRUCTION

Charles Woods and Noah Wason

Wearable devices are digital technologies designed to be worn on the body and include products like FitBit, smart earphones, and smartwatches. These products change how many people do their jobs: how athletes compete, musicians compose, and coworkers communicate. They also change the relationship these users have with data. Recently, Big Technology (Big Tech) companies like Apple, Google, and Meta (Facebook) have expanded their advertising and marketing campaigns to amplify health-related devices and applications (apps). While these companies are explicit in how these products and services can be valuable to users, the privacy information they provide users is markedly vague. Wearable technologies that collect biometric information have the potential to change the way users interact with their health data and by extension their doctors and other health care professionals. With the proliferation of wearable technologies and the increasing call for on-demand health information following the COVID-19 pandemic, users and health care professionals must be more attentive to privacy issues concerning wearable technologies.

On September 14, 2021, Apple Inc. (Apple) released a promotional video advertisement for the Apple Watch Series 7, a new product in the Apple Watch line that debuted in 2015. In addition to depicting various Apple product "users" engaged in numerous athletic activities, the promotional video also details the exciting new digital tracking capabilities of the wearable device: the speed of a tennis serve, the distance of a golf drive, the number of waves ridden on a surfboard, but also a user's pulse, blood oxygen level, electro-cardiograms, and sleep patterns. The video ends on an ostentatious promise to users: "The future of health is on your wrist." While this ambitious future encourages user agency and access to personal health-related data, it also presumes a certain level of health

DOI: 10.4324/9781003316770-14

literacy among users. Unfortunately, the average user may not understand the long-term implications of these technologies.

Apple forecasted these new device features in its December 2020, privacy policy update, the first update to their policy following the Apple Watch Series 6 release in September 2020. While Apple robustly explains the types of data they collect in other sections of their Terms of Service (ToS) documents, the December 2020 policy is the first time the company mentions "health information" specifically in the privacy policy:

> **Health Information:** Data relating to the health status of an individual, including data related to one's physical or mental health or condition. Personal health data also includes data that can be used to make inferences about or detect the health status of an individual. If you participate in a study using an Apple Health Research Study app, the policy governing the privacy of your personal data is described in the Apple Health Study Apps Privacy Policy. (n.p.)

In addition to broadly defining "health information" as anything related to physical and mental health, Apple's privacy policy fails to mention the nuances of its collection, aggregation, and use of data. More pointedly: how many everyday users can actually explain how the data wearable devices collect "can be used to make inferences about or detect the health status of an individual"? What the privacy policy for Apple makes clear is that health literacies must now (but do not yet) include data literacies. In this chapter, we analyze the Apple Watch Series 7 privacy policy, highlight ideas for intervention, and discuss the implications for undergraduate writing instruction (UWI). Ultimately, we argue for a convergence between health literacies and data literacies among users of wearable technologies.

Locating Data and Health Literacies

Revised definitions for understanding health literacies from Healthy People 2030, the United States Department of Health and Human Services (HSS) decade-long campaign for addressing critical health issues in the country, focus on people's ability to make "well-informed" instead of "appropriate" decisions. These definitions suggest people move beyond just understanding this information to *using* it in their everyday routines. Additionally, HSS's updated definitions of "personal health literacy" and "organizational health literacy" now include perspectives from the larger public and express the responsibility of organizations to specifically address the topic of health literacies. In creating dual definitions for individuals and for organizations, HSS has started to acknowledge that average Americans are increasingly collecting and using their personal health data and rely on Big Tech companies to provide them with the means to do so.

Privacy policies for wearable devices that collect health data are a site where information about personal health literacies, organizational health literacies, and understanding the nuances of digital privacy converge. Data collecting wearable devices inherently change a user's relationship to data, and given the ever-increasing likelihood that users will incorporate these devices into their health and wellness regimen, privacy policies become more than ToS documents: they potentially become patient materials. The Agency for Healthcare Research and Quality (AHRQ) suggests health care professionals (and by extension, undergraduate writing instructors who teach future health care professionals) focus on providing patients with "understandable" materials which consider elements like "word choice, organization of information, [and] formatting" alongside general readability (p. 35). The goal is to ensure that patients can acquire and comprehend health-related information enough to make "appropriate" health decisions (p. 1). Privacy policies are not written with these same intentions in mind despite the fact that Big Tech companies fully intend for their wearable devices to collect personal health-related information from users.

As important legal documents, privacy policies typically address what data companies collect from users and how they can use this data for various purposes. To Apple's credit, their privacy policy is easy for users to navigate: the digital document includes a series of hyperlinks near the beginning that allows them to navigate to the sections of the policy they want to read, including information related to how health data is collected and used. Hyperlinks to supplemental information are also embedded throughout the text. Apple's privacy policy includes an opt-in feature, a best practice that allows users to decide if they want to access all of Apple's products and services and share the requisite data. In order to focus user attention, Apple makes good use of bolded fonts in its privacy policy to amplify information beyond headings and subheadings that users might otherwise overlook. For example, in the privacy policy section titled "Cookies and Other Technologies," Apple emphasizes the following: "These technologies help us to better understand user behavior including security and fraud prevention purposes, tell us which parts of our websites people have visited, and facilitate and measure the effectiveness of advertising and web searches" (Apple, 2022). In this moment of transparency, Apple directs user attention to how cookies and other tracking technologies are used and why.

While Apple's privacy policy is well-designed and readable, that does not mean it aids user comprehension of the actual terms of service for their devices or what the company could do with the health information it collects. Due to their focus on "patient experience and improving the design of information," undergraduate writing instructors with expertise in the rhetorics of health and medicine may be uniquely positioned to help improve materials in ways that both cater to patient needs and helps them understand their personal health information (Melonçon & Frost, 2015, pp. 7–11). Moreover, centering the patient experience means navigating the interpersonal relationships between health care professionals and the patients who rely on their expertise.

Wearable devices potentially change the relationship between patients and health care providers. The proliferation of wearable technologies that record health information is not the first time that this relationship has been altered. The onset of digital discussion spaces (i.e., Facebook groups, online forums, etc.) has already shifted how users search for and understand health-related information in ways that health care providers haven't always been able to address (Gurak, 2018, pp. 127–128). Similar to the features designed for medical wearables, digital writing spaces afford users a different level of interactivity than a traditional health care provider. In a sense, users' trust in the expertise of their health care provider might be mediated through a larger ecology that now includes other patients and digital technologies. Devices like the Apple Watch Series 7 seem to give users even more agency over their health information and decision-making, but by further altering their relationship with an important part of their healthcare ecology (health care providers), these devices may change a patient's comprehension of their own health information.

The Apple Watch Series 7 promises users a reliable means for generating their own health data thereby creating an additional source of medical information. The health data generated by wearable devices should be considered ancillary by users, and yet Apple's advertising encourages users to incorporate the device as a primary source of health information. Health care providers subsequently become but one source of information amongst many others, further emphasizing that health literacies are a shared set of practices (Paakkari & Okan, 2020). Furthermore, the need to consult a multitude of health information sources exacerbates what is already a complex undertaking. Only 12% of U.S. adults have the health literacy skills needed to manage the demands of the complex American healthcare system, and their ability to absorb and use health information can be compromised by stress or illness (AHRQ, 2020).

Adding on the privacy policies required for medical wearables makes it even less likely that users will develop the health literacies required to make well-informed decisions. Many Americans understand that companies are collecting data from them every day; however, they also maintain various emotions about digital privacy and security, including confusion and concern about a lack of control (Pew, 2019). To encourage well-informed decisions regarding medical wearables, we suggest addressing issues like transparency and data usage in privacy policies because these kinds of analyses can reveal important intersections between digital privacy and health literacies.

Understanding Two Concepts: Transparency and Data Usage

As early as 2010, Big Tech companies (e.g., Google, Apple) have offered documents called "transparency reports" that share how government and corporate policies impact digital privacy, security, and access. While transparency reports provide users with a brief glimpse into a company's compliance procedures, they are not themselves meaningful explanations of the ToS users agree to in privacy policies. Moving towards user-centered privacy policies for wearable devices requires what Darwish (2008) describes as transparency "determined by the reader's ability to analyze the text and process information and by the shared knowledge and intersubjectivity between writer (as conveyed by the text) and reader" (p. 155-56). Therefore, a policy is only "transparent" if users can understand the information in a way that lets them make informed decisions.

Transparency remains complex because many technology companies are intentionally ambiguous about their methods of data collection and use. Indeed, the commodification of user data is what fuels the internet, so there is not much incentive for Big Tech companies whose products already flood the market to be transparent. When we consent to a privacy policy, it is not a completely "informed" decision. It's like being sent an invitation to a party by someone you know, but the invitation lacks information about the time and location of the event. Furthermore, the party organizer is going to send a car for you to take you to the party, but you have to be blindfolded for the duration of your ride. In this analogy, the party organizer clearly knows who you are and where you live, but this information is not reciprocal. Overcoming the lack of transparency requires a great deal of trust in the party organizer. How many of us would get into a car blindfolded to attend an event without knowing the route and destination? How many of us would then sign a contract accepting a laundry list of terms and conditions absolving the party organizer of responsibility for any harm? And yet, this is what we do every time we consent to a privacy policy. We are promised a transformative device or service, and we must trust all of its processes are not only benign but necessary.

The unique thing about wearable technologies like the Apple Watch is that they now provide users with access to sensitive health information. More recent privacy policies better emphasize that data collection happens (e.g., Apple's previously mentioned use of bolded fonts to draw user attention to tracking technologies). These policies are designed to build a sense of trust with users that the data collection powering these devices is in their best interest; however, they rarely clarify the exact mechanisms for collecting and utilizing this personal information. For instance, Apple Watch users have some autonomy over what information they share, but Apple ultimately decides what personal data and metadata (i.e., geolocation) are valuable enough to pool together for third-party partners like advertisers. Data collection, then, is like being on an elevator with someone who knows everything about you (Apple, Facebook, Google) and then proceeds to whisper an elevator pitch about you to every individual who gets on the elevator (third parties). You do not get to choose the content of the pitch, and companies like Apple do not disclose what they said to other elevator passengers. Now imagine this elevator pitch includes your sensitive medical information and an insurance agent is one of the elevator passengers.

As it pertains to Apple's Privacy Policy, transparency requires attention to specific policy updates including data collection methods and usage (Woods & Wason, 2021). The Apple Watch collects various biometric data from users (e.g., heart rate, oxygen level, blood pressure, walking speed, etc.) in order to provide the promised health data related to various physical activities (e.g., biking, hiking, sleeping, etc). As previously mentioned, Apple made substantial changes to its privacy policy in December 2020 to account for the new capabilities of its devices; however, these alterations are far from transparent for everyday users and health care professionals because Apple does not make a database of former policies readily available. In the following section, we analyze the Apple Privacy Policy updated June 1, 2021, as an illustrative example with specific attention to transparency and data usage.

Analysis of Apple's Privacy Policy

Many of the issues with transparency in the privacy policy for Apple products begin with their lack of specificity concerning what counts as health information. While these policies are written in simple language in comparison to the jargon-ridden legalese one might expect, they do not actually provide users with additional clarity. As the "Health Information" portion of their "Personal Data Apple Collects from You" section details, Apple's definition of "personal health data" specifically includes "data that can be used to make inferences about or detect the health status of an individual" (Apple, 2022). Arguably, Apple's definition of health information is so broad that it could encapsulate any data Apple unilaterally decides is related to a user's health status. Apple maintains flexibility by keeping their definition vague, thus providing itself substantial latitude for collecting various information that users and doctors would not readily consider health information.

Lack of transparency includes broad definitions, but it also includes creating obstacles to information like burying it in other documents that are only accessible via hyperlink. Users who desire to learn more precisely how Apple uses their health data (or their data in general) must follow a hyperlink to a "Data and Privacy" page which lists *over 70* different data policies for various Apple products and services, any number of which could be used in conjunction with Apple Watch Series 7. Currently, there are six policies hyperlinked on the "Data and Privacy" page that we consider directly related to health information (as it pertains to the Apple Watch Series 7). Each one is a distinct policy and varies in length: "Health App & Privacy"; "Health Records & Privacy"; "Improve Health and Activity & Privacy"; "Improve Health Records & Privacy"; "Apple Fitness+ & Privacy"; "Improve Fitness+ & Privacy." Forcing users to click a hyperlink (or even a series of hyperlinks) and then sift through information provided across multiple documents is an inconsiderate practice at best and a deceptive one at worst, particularly when it obscures information from users who wish to make meaningful, informed decisions.

For example, under their "Health App & Privacy" policy, Apple states users have control over the information shared with their health app including what information is added and how long it is retained in the cloud. However, to even learn that they are sharing information, users need to consult yet another hyperlink to yet another webpage. While not a rabbit hole, it is certainly a goose chase for users. You have access to policies, but it's hard to understand them because the specifics are all over the place. In having to consult all these different documents, it is hard to form a cohesive sense of what is important.

Data usage concerns how companies like Apple and third-party applications and services utilize data collected from users. Unfortunately, Apple's privacy policy really only provides information about how data are collected, leaving users with only half of the information needed to understand where their data goes and how it is used once it is collected. For example, the Series 7 Watch collects health information like user heart rate, but it also collects usage data such as browsing history and location data in the form of geo-tagging. What does heart rate have to do with browsing history and location? The answer is unclear, and yet between the Series 7 Watch and the iPhone required for it to function, Apple collects all three (and without explaining the different uses of this data).

Users have a vested interest in how their personal data is used and its legal and ethical implications, but so does Apple. The company establishes a wide purview for operationalizing user data in moments it defines as of "legitimate interest" but Apple's privacy policy does not define what this means:

> We may also process your personal data where we believe it is in our or others legitimate interests, taking into consideration your interests, rights, and expectations. If you have questions about the legal basis, you can contact the Data Protection Officer at apple.com/legal/privacy/contact. (n.p.)

In writing its privacy policy in this way, Apple once again places the responsibility on users to thoroughly investigate critical information that Apple clearly knows, but does not share transparently. Whereas patients can directly ask (or even call) their primary physicians, Apple does not facilitate direct human-to-human interaction. Instead, users can only submit an online form.

The interface for communicating with Apple officials does very little to guide inquiry as it assumes users already have specific questions and/or knowledge about what they are asking. To initiate a request, users must fill out an online "Privacy Inquiries" form that imitates an email to the company consisting of their specific question(s) and personal contact information (e.g., name, email address). This rudimentary form is a stark contrast to the sound design of their privacy policy because it fails to provide users with any assistance in formulating their questions (e.g., prompts or examples for the kinds of inquiries users have made). If the user does not already know what questions to ask about their privacy, the form is useless. Additionally, unlike a personal physician, Apple does not give a sense of who the Data Protection Officer is (even though the Data Protection Officer is referenced in the policy). The interface is also not designed to guide users in developing their inquiry (e.g., what evidence or explanations to include) nor does it provide any information related to the inquiry submission review process (e.g., how long it typically takes to receive a response). As with their "Personal Data Apple Collects From You" section, Apple only provides vague and/or incomplete definitions and obstacles (i.e., the inquiry submission form) that prevent users from efficiently acquiring additional information.

Apple's Privacy Policy is careful not to mandate users share data, but they are also clear that users cannot access products and services without consent:

> You are not required to provide the personal data that we have requested. However, if you choose not to do so, in many cases we will not be able to provide you with products or services or respond to requests you may have. (n.p.)

This creates a situation where consumers can only use devices and services they paid for if they are willing to also share all of the data Apple requests. Quite literally, these devices only work if users opt to share their data. If Apple were truly transparent, such caveats would be included in their advertisements. Further complicating matters are third-party app developers which Apple requires to have their own separate policies. As Apple explains in their separate "Health Apps & Privacy" document, "Each app is also required to have a privacy policy that describes its use of health data, so you [users] should review these policies before providing apps with access to your health data." Apple acknowledges that numerous developers are interested in users' personal health information, but it places the responsibility on users to protect this information themselves. Apple assumes that most users have the data literacies necessary to understand what information they would be surrendering to developers; they also assume that users comprehend the long-term effects of adopting these third-party applications.

Discussion and Extensions

Provided Apple does not highlight policy changes for users, we argue that attention to transparency and data usage are critical starting points for students engaging with those policies. Undergraduate writing instructors and their students must consider the critical intersection of digital privacy and the collection of health-related data – especially when the very use of these technologies require a significant level of opting into data collection, even if users do not fully understand what they are consenting to. As previously mentioned, Apple ends the "Personal Data Apple Collects from You" section of their privacy policy with a catch-22: if users don't share data they cannot access services they pay for (which includes devices like the Apple Watch Series 7). Undergraduate writing instructors and their students must push for transparency regarding health-related information from companies that sell these technologies. Where does the data go once it is collected and aggregated? Who owns the data collected from wearable devices? What are the third-parties Apple is working with, and what data does Apple provide them access to? This is but a small sampling of the critical questions researches in health-related fields need to raise.

There are many ways to go about answering the aforementioned questions, including continuing research related to wearable devices like the Apple Watch Series 7 and similar technologies. Writing instructors can also survey and perform research studies that focus on the needs of medical practitioners including information about the impact wearable devices have on their work and the work of other professionals in the field. They can create course assignments, classroom activities, and/or entire units of their writing courses with the explicit purpose of teaching students about digital security as a critical aspect of patient wellbeing.

Relatedly, writing instructors can incorporate health information assignments into their regular instruction. For instance, instructors teaching first-year composition (FYC), technical and professional communication, and digital rhetorics as a part of UWI can discuss the privacy policies for health-related technologies and the ways these documents could potentially disrupt relationships between health care providers and their patients. Students in these courses can also discuss the larger implications for further entrenching technology into our private lives to reveal systemic social inequity and identify ubiquitous surveillance practices. These conversations can address issues such as inequities in technological device access across users from different socioeconomic backgrounds, the racial dynamics of provider and patient relationships, and the narrow set of user experiences that device features are designed towards.

While the focus of this chapter is on how undergraduate writing instructors can engage their students with issues at the intersection of digital privacy and health literacies, these complex issues require an interdisciplinary approach. Engineering students interested in designing wearable technologies (like the Apple Watch Series 7) would benefit from these courses, and Kirk St. Amant's approach, detailed in the next chapter, can provide a useful guide. There is additional potential for classrooms that develop a coalition of viewpoints from various disciplines. For example, assignments that ask students to speculate about future devices that utilize health data (e.g., wearables that automatically share vitals related to COVID-19) would certainly encourage students to think about the intersections between the health and Big Tech industries. A "health literacies across the curriculum" approach may be helpful (see Chapter 8).

There is an emergent need to develop innovative digital technologies that provide health-related information to governments at local, state, and national levels in order to make large-scale, informed decisions related to public health policy. This is already happening in states like New York where health departments are releasing their own smartphone applications to assist residents with COVID-19-related reporting and notifications. The New York State Department of Health provides the "COVID Alter NY" application on both the Apple App Store and Google Play Store. This app alerts users when they have been within six feet of someone with coronavirus for more than 10 minutes; anonymously notifies others if they were in contact with you while reporting symptoms; and allows you to keep a private log of your own symptoms (NY Health, 2021). Vaccine passports are another example of an emerging technology that allows people to securely store their vaccine status on their devices. Provided governments have already considered using vaccine passports as a way to limit the spread of COVID-19 through travel (British Broadcasting Corporation, 2021), studying this documentation can help scholars think about border crossing, medical misinformation, and patient access to vaccine status (some of which may be granted through third-party companies). These inquiries immediately highlight the same issues of access, transparency, and consent we have investigated with the Apple Watch Series 7 in this chapter.

Ultimately, undergraduate writing courses that inspect how health information is collected and used can help students to consider how much data contributes to otherwise routine medical decision-making (regular doctor visits, workout regimes, etc.). Whether we want it to or not, data now factors into our decision-making at every level, from the personal (or local) level to global public health crises. Understanding health information and making well-informed decisions requires acknowledging the ways digital surveillance has infiltrated what may otherwise seem like mundane, inconsequential aspects of our lived experience.

Conclusion

Apple is not being hyperbolic when they claim, "The future of health is on your wrist." As explored in this chapter, the future of health information in UWI requires attention to medical wearables and the companies that produce them, the systems that make them possible, and the policies that govern their use. Investigations into wearables that collect and use health-related information should begin with privacy policies themselves. While we investigate the privacy policy for the Apple Watch Series 7, there are similar policies for various data-collecting wearable devices that many health care providers are already familiar with: hearing aids, glucose monitors, insulin pumps, etc. In future studies, researchers might examine how different iterations of the Starkey Evolv AI Hearing aid sports utilizes artificially intelligent systems to make automatic adjustments or how the Dexcom G6 CGM shares data with the Tandem Diabetes Care T:slim X2 Control-IQ Pump to monitor glucose levels and allow patients to share their health-data with caregivers and family through an associated app.

Students in undergraduate writing courses can learn a great deal about how writing influences the healthcare ecosystem. As more people adopt consumer-grade digital technologies to record their personal health information, the required literacies will change, too. In this chapter, we considered issues with transparency and data collection with the Apple Watch Series 7; however, these are not the only issues that students in undergraduate writing courses should be familiar with when examining privacy policies and other ToS documents. For example, there are other issues involving temporality (e.g., when the policy was published and updated) and specific tracking technologies (e.g., cookies, SDKs) that monitor and record user activity (Woods & Wason, 2021). In working through assignments that delve into data usage, undergraduate students can learn how data impacts their interactions in both digital spaces and physical spaces – within and beyond formal healthcare settings.

References

Agency for Healthcare Research and Quality. (2020). *Health literacy university precautions toolkit* (2nd Ed.). Washington, D.C.: Agency for Healthcare Research and Quality. Available at: http://www.ahrq.gov/literacy

Apple, Inc. (2022). *Apple privacy policy.* https://www.apple.com/legal/privacy/en-ww/.

Auxier, B., Rainie, L., Anderson, M., Perrin, A., Kumar, M., & Turner, E. (2019, November 15). Americans and privacy: Concerned, confused, and feeling lack of control over their personal information. *Pew Research Center.* https://www.pewresearch.org/internet/2019/11/15/americans-and-privacy-concerned-confused-and-feeling-lack-of-control-over-their-personal-information/

British Broadcasting Corporation. (2021, April 4). *Vaccine passport: What is it and why are people talking about it?* https://www.bbc.co.uk/newsround/56520612

Darwish, A. (2008). *Optimality in translation.* Victoria, Canada: Writescope.

Gurak, L. J. (2018). Ethos, trust, and the rhetoric of digital writing in scientific and technical discourse. In J. Alexander & J. Rhodes (Eds.), *The Routledge handbook of digital writing and rhetoric* (pp. 124–131). London: Routledge.

Melonçon, L., & Frost, E. A. (2015). Charting an emerging field: The rhetoric of health and medicine and its importance in communication design. *Communication Design Quarterly,* 3(4), 7–14.

NY Health. (2021). *Covid alert NY: What you need to know.* https://coronavirus.health.ny.gov/covid-alert-ny-what-you-need-know

Paakkari, L., & Okan, O. (2020). COVID-19: Health literacy is an underestimated problem. *The Lancet Public Health*, 5(5), e249–e250. 10.1016/S2468-2667(20)30086-4

United States Department of Health and Human Services. (n.d.). *Health Literacy in Health People 2030*. https://health.gov/healthypeople/priority-areas/health-literacy-healthy-people-2030

Woods, C., & Wason, N. (2021). The rhetorical implications of data aggregation: becoming a 'dividual' in a data-driven world. *The Journal of Interactive Technology and Pedagogy*. https://jitp.commons.gc.cuny.edu/category/issues/issue-nineteen/

11

CREATING CONTENT FOR CONTEXTS OF CARE: A COGNITIVE APPROACH TO ACHIEVING HEALTH LITERACIES THROUGH USABILITY

Kirk St.Amant

According to current definitions, health literacy involves more than if individuals can understand the information presented in a document, image, or other communication resources. Now, a core – and increasingly primary – element of health literacies involves usability, or if individuals can act on, or use, information to achieve a health-related objective (health.gov, 2021; World Health Organization, 2022). However, what constitutes usability within health literacies is not universal. Rather, expectations of usability often reflect pre-existing mental models of what individuals expect to occur in a healthcare context. Such expectations encompass the locations where individuals can access healthcare services, the person who provide such services, and the items those persons use to provide care (St.Amant, 2017 & 2019a). If communicators in the healthcare industry understand these factors, they can design materials that meet the usability needs of different audiences (Melonçon, 2017; St.Amant, 2019a). The complexities of these situations are considerable, yet addressing them is key to meeting the health literacy needs of different audiences. Prototype theory can help in addressing such dynamics.

Prototype theory focuses on how individuals recognize locations, persons, and items. As such, it can help identify the variables influencing usability expectations and affecting literacy factors in healthcare contexts (Melonçon, 2017; St.Amant, 2017). Specifically, prototype theory can provide a framework for understanding the usability expectations central to health literacies in different situations. This chapter explains how to apply prototype theory to address an audience's usability and associated literacy expectations and needs in different healthcare contexts. Because of its flexibility, prototype theory can be adapted for various assignments, courses, and programs related to undergraduate writing instruction.

DOI: 10.4324/9781003316770-15

Usability in Health Literacies

Addressing health literacies focuses on creating materials for sharing health and medical information effectively with different audiences (Melonçon, 2017). These processes involve content, or materials used to convey ideas. In some cases, this content is verbal (usually written text); in others, it is visual (e.g., images, charts, etc.), a theme discussed in other chapters in this collection. Moreover, organizations often combine both kinds of content to convey ideas according to the health literacy needs of audiences (Heifferon, 2004).

Historically, such processes have been guided by patient literacy and understanding how the background of the patients affects the usability of content (Heifferon, 2004; Melonçon, 2017).

Addressing such factors often focused on the register, vocabulary, tone, and style used to present concepts. While this focus contributed to texts audiences could understand, it did not necessarily mean that such texts were usable. Rather, the location where individuals performed activities affected the usability of content as much as the ability of individuals to recognize images and understand texts (St.Amant, 2019a).

Where one performs an activity affects what one can do. Administering an injection in a well-lit, quiet setting like one's living room is one thing; doing so in a dimly lit, busy train en route to work is another (St.Amant, 2019a & b). These environmental factors affect how individuals achieve the same objective (administering an injection) in different contexts (St.Amant, 2017). In other cases, certain technologies might be central to performing a care-related activity, and again, factors of location can affect such processes. Individuals, for example, might need to plug in a device, access the Internet, or call an outside party as a part of a healthcare activity. If power, online access, or phone services are not available in a location, then content based on such factors is of limited use. In such situations, healthcare content needs revision to address such contextual differences and allow individuals to achieve healthcare objectives in such settings (St.Amant, 2019b). In this way, understanding and addressing the context where audiences use content is central to achieving effective health literacies.

Understanding Usability

The term "usability" generally means how easily individuals can "use" an item to achieve an objective (Interaction Design Foundation, n. d.). The objective of using a stethoscope, for example, might be to listen to someone's heartbeat. The "usability" of that stethoscope, however, involves how easily individuals can use that stethoscope to achieve this objective. The relationship to between usability and ease of achieving an objective has three core parts:

- *Identification:* individuals using an item can readily identify it (e.g., item is a stethoscope).

- *Operation:* individuals know what an item does and how to use it to perform those processes (e.g., knows stethoscopes let one listen to sounds produced inside of something).
- *Contextualization:* items can do multiple things; the appropriate use reflects where individuals use an item (e.g., in a medical context, use a stethoscope to check a heartbeat vs. an engine) (St.Amant, 2018a).

When individuals encounter items, they must perform all three processes to use items effectively in order to achieve a desired objective (i.e., the reason for which they are in a given setting).

These processes do not occur simultaneously. Rather, it is a cascading effect where an initial stimulus, or trigger, starts one process that then initiates the next process that initiates the third (Eyal, 2014; Lindstrom, 2010). This triggered-cascade generally works in one of two ways:

- *Object Triggering:* the cascade starts when an individual identifies an object. Upon recognizing an object (initiates or triggers a cascade), that person then accesses a mental association for what that item does and how it is used to perform different processes. (This is why individuals often know what at item does once they recognize it.) Next, the individual notes the location in which the item appears to determine the appropriate use of that item.
- *Place Triggering:* this process begins when individuals survey their surroundings to identify where they are. The identification of the location then triggers expectations of the actions that should occur in that setting and associated items use to perform those activities. Individuals, for example, generally go to a hospital emergency room to receive care (objective). They often expect the emergency room they visit to have a computer used to "check patients in," and they expect to provide the user of that computer with information (e.g., name, address, insurance) for this process. In this way, place triggers expectations of what items individuals will encounter and use in a location to perform the activities associated with that setting. (For more examples – and possible complications – see Chapter 9, where Katherine E. Morelli discusses the work of cultural health navigators.)

In both cases, identification initiates the cascade process and involves similar cognitive factors: *prototypes*, or mental models for the design and function of items (St.Amant, 2018b).

Cognition of Recognition

All individuals have mental models for what characteristics certain items should have in order to recognize them. This representation springs to mind when individuals hear or read a particular word. This mental model is a *prototype*

(Aitchison, 1994; Rosch, 1978). Individuals encounter the word "scalpel," for example, a prototype (mental depiction) of a small, stainless steel cutting tool with a razor-sharp end comes to mind. Prototypes consist of two kinds of features, or characteristics:

- *Sensory characteristics:* the expectations individuals have for what something should look, feel, sound, smell, or taste like in order to recognize it (e.g., a scalpel is a small, stainless steel object with a razor-sharp end).
- *Attributional characteristics:* the functions or actions individuals associate with that item/what the item can do (e.g., a scalpel is used for cutting during medical procedures) (Aitchison, 1994; Rosch, 1978).

So, when an individual encounter the word "syringe," that person's mind accesses a mental model, or prototype, noting sensory characteristics like a syringe is cylindrical and of a size that fits in a closed hand. This prototype also includes the attributional characteristics that individuals use syringes to inject substances into things, like the body. Similarly, when one encounters the word "physician," a mental model of a person in a white coat (sensory characteristic) who does certain things to assess one's health (attributional characteristic) comes to mind. These mental models are *object prototypes* associated with specific items or persons – what objects or individuals are and what they do (St.Amant, 2018b; Lindstrom, 2010).

The same process works for places. When individuals encounter the term "examination room," a model pops to mind including what that room looks like (e.g., what is in it), smells like, sounds like, and feels like (e.g., scent of antiseptic, cold floors, and humming of overhead lights).

Likewise, this mental model brings attributional expectations of what processes individuals expect to occur there (e.g., medical processes). This mental model also notes who will perform these processes (e.g., trained medical professionals), and what those individuals will use to perform those processes (e.g., with a stethoscope and blood pressure cuff). This mental model for a location is a *prototype of place* – a mental representation individuals use to identify locations and the activities performed there (St.Amant, 2018b; Lindstrom, 2010). Both kinds of prototype operate according to identification based on sensory features, and these processes often work in one of two ways (Aitchison, 1994; Lindstrom, 2010; St.Amant, 2018b).

When an individual hears or reads the word "stethoscope," a mental model (prototype) pops in the mind of what a stethoscope looks like, feels, like, sounds like, etc. If someone asks the individual to locate a "stethoscope," that person's mind accesses this prototype, and that individual then searches the surrounding location for something that resembles that prototype (Wolfe, 1994 & 2007).

The same processes work for prototypes of place (St.Amant, 2018b). If individuals know they are searching for an "examining room," their minds access the prototype they have for what an examining room looks, sounds, smells, feels, and tastes like. They then use that model to search for the related place (i.e., an examining room). If individuals don't know where they are, they review the features in their surroundings to determine how many of these features match the prototypes they have for different locations. Individuals will continue this process until they have a prototype of place match and know where they are. After identifying the location, the individual's mind accesses the associated actions to perform in that location, and they then initiate the related process – including noting objects to look for and use in that setting.

In these processes, object prototypes and prototypes of place are connected. When individuals scan their environment to look for features that identify where they are, they use object prototypes to identify these features/characteristics (e.g., a check-in desk in an emergency room) (St.Amant, 2018b). If individuals can identify enough features/characteristics to mirror their prototype expectations for a particular location, they can recognize where they are. Conversely, if in-dividuals know where they are, the associated prototype of place brings ex-pectations of items they expect to encounter there and what features these items should have so individuals can recognize and use them. The prototype of place for "emergency room," for example, brings the expectation a "check-in desk" and "chairs" should be there as well as what that desk and these chairs should look, feel like, etc.

Creating Prototypes

Prototypes are not inherent to humans. Rather, individuals develop them over time based on exposure to various stimuli (Aitchison, 1994; Rosch, 1978). This process can create different expectations for how individuals identify and use items or interact with individuals in healthcare contexts (St.Amant, 2017).

The first time individuals encounter an object, they rely on those around them to identify that object by giving it a "name." Usually, someone shows the in-dividual an object and then says the name of that item. ("This is a Band-Aid™.") Individuals then note what the item looks like as well as the term associated with it. Over time, individuals will encounter other kinds of Band-Aids™ and realize, while differences might occur (e.g., color and shape), certain features are common across all versions (sterile padding and adhesive on one side, non-stick on the other). Through this continued exposure and comparison, individuals fine-tune the prototype for "Band-Aid™" to note an object must have these characteristics to be a Band-Aid™ (Aitchison, 1994). They then use this prototype to identify Band-Aids™ in their environment.

The same process influences how individuals learn prototypes for place (St.Amant, 2018b). The first time an individual enters a healthcare context, someone often identifies that context for them, such as noting the individual is about to enter the "examining room." Once in that location, the individual surveys that setting and notes the features that seem unique to that location and set it apart from other known locations. In an examining room, individuals might note the table that can sit up or recline; they might also notice a counter lined with canisters of cotton swabs, tongue depressors, and cotton balls. Accordingly, the more individuals visit the same kind of location, the more they establish the items they commonly encounter in that setting. Over time, these items become the characteristics individuals expect to encounter and use to identify that location.

Because prototypes reflect experience, different experiences can lead to the creation of different prototypes for objects or locations (St.Amant, 2017 & 2018b). Varied life experiences could mean individuals associate different prototypes with the same term (Aitchison, 1994; Rosch, 1978). When I, for example, encounter the term "blood pressure cuff," a mental image of an automated band placed around the wrist might pop to mind (i.e., a digital blood pressure cuff). You, however, might think of a band that goes around the upper arm and uses a circular gauge to measure pressure – as well as has a "pump" attachment for inflating the cuff (i.e., a manual blood pressure cuff). This factor affects how each of us recognizes and uses a "blood pressure cuff" to check our blood pressure.

Similarly, we might associate different locations with the same healthcare process (St.Amant, 2019b). We might both check our blood pressure daily. I do it at the end of the day on the train ride home from work while surrounded by numerous individuals, sights, sounds, etc., as I use an automated device to check my blood pressure myself. You, however, might have your partner use a stethoscope and a manual blood pressure cuff to check your blood pressure while sitting at your kitchen table in the relative calm of the early morning. These different scenarios affect how we think about and perform the same care-related activity.

As such, variations in experiences can create usability problems (St.Amant, 2019a & b). If I am accustomed to using one kind of blood pressure cuff, I might not know what features to look for or how to use a different design. I might also use that other version incorrectly and get an inaccurate reading that prompts me to think I have a condition (e.g., low blood pressure). Similarly, if I am accustomed to performing this process in a different location, I might assume I can use certain items that might not be present (e.g., someone will provide an analog blood pressure cuff or there will be a power outlet for using a digital one). As a result, I might not know how to use a device I am familiar with in a different context. Such prototype-based differences have important implications for health literacies in terms of creating texts, images, and other kinds of content audiences can use to effectively perform healthcare activities.

Expectations and Errors

When creating health-related content, differences in prototype expectations become particularly problematic due to *default assumptions* (Eyal, 2014; St.Amant, 2017). A default assumption involves thinking one's own experiences are commonplace and defaulting to the assumption others do things the same way (St.Amant, 2019a). If I use a battery-powered digital cuff to monitor my blood pressure, my default assumption is others use the same technology for this process.

These default assumptions affect how individuals conceptualize ideas to share with others. The content-creation process generally begins with authors or designers accessing a mental model of the process they wish to convey (Eyal, 2014; Lindstrom, 2010). This model is often akin to a movie scene in which an individual performs the activity in a particular location using specific objects and sometimes interacting with other individuals during this process. Using this model as a guide, content creators describe in writing or depict in images the scenes playing out in their minds (Eyal, 2014; Lindstrom, 2010). The objective is to create a text or an image that encapsulates what occurs in that scene (mental modal) in order to provide the information needed for others to re-create this process – or replicate this scene – when readers or viewers undertake the same activity.

These default assumptions involve the prototype of the place content creators have for where they experienced the related process (St.Amant, 2018b). Within these prototypes of place are object prototypes: items the audience expects to find and use in that location in order to perform the related process there. Yet, the content creator's experiences are not inherently the same as the audiences who will use health or medical content (St.Amant, 2018b). Rather, prospective dis-connects resulting from different prototype associations for locations or objects can affect the usability of healthcare content.

The audiences reading or viewing such content might use different items (object prototype) to perform an activity (St.Amant, 2017 & 2019a). Per the blood pressure example, individuals using my instructions might not have access to a digital blood pressure cuff, but instead use a stethoscope and a manual blood pressure cuff to check their blood pressure. This disconnect in object prototypes means that audience cannot use my content, for it describes a process involving the use of a different technology to achieve a healthcare objective (St.Amant, 2017 & 2019a). Even if content creator and audience associate the same location with an activity, differences in items essential to performing a process can limit the usability of content.

Both content creator and audience could associate the location of "one's living room" with where to check blood pressure. If, however, each party expects to use a different item to perform this process in that location, then performing the related process becomes an issue. In these ways, default assumptions can affect the usability of healthcare content even when activities take place in a common location.

In other cases, differing prototypes of place can affect the usability of health or medical content (St.Amant, 2017 & 2019a). I might assume my experiences checking my blood sugar levels when sitting quietly in my personal office re-presents the scenario to document when creating content on how to perform this process. As a result, I create instructional content according to the dynamics of this location (my default prototype of place for this activity). The audience who uses this content, however, might perform this activity in a different setting – like the kitchen of their home while watching their children at the end of the day. This setting brings different expectations of the user's ability to maintain focus on the content provided given what is occurring in that environment at that time. Such a difference could affect how individuals use the content I created to perform this process in that environment.

In both cases, default assumptions for prototypes affect the usability of healthcare content. For these reasons, individuals such as Melonçon (2016 & 2017), Agboka (2014), and Saru and Wojan (2020) advocated a usability-focused approach to creating health-related materials for audiences. This approach requires an understanding of where individuals use information and the items they have access to in that location. To do so, content creators need to identify the contexts audiences associate with healthcare activities, for addressing such dynamics is central to meeting the health literacy needs of different groups (Acharya, 2019; Melonçon, 2017).

Researching Prototype Expectations

According to prototype theory, individuals cannot assume their conceptualization of locations or objects is universal (Aitchison, 1994; St.Amant, 2015). To address this factor, the creators of healthcare content need to do more than research an audience's background (e.g., education level, familiarity with topic, etc.) (Melonçon, 2017; St.Amant, 2017). They also need to identify the prototypes these individuals rely on when using informational and instructional materials (St.Amant, 2015). Gaining such understanding involves interacting with audiences to gather information on the prototypes they associate with healthcare contexts (Melonçon, 2017; St.Amant, 2017).

Essentially, individuals from certain backgrounds and from certain locations often have common experiences interacting with healthcare services (Heifferon, 2004; Melonçon, 2017; St.Amant, 2019a). For this reason, researching such factors should begin by identifying the audience that will use healthcare content. Factors to consider include not only demographic, educational, and socio-economic information, but also

- Healthcare services available in the community (including clinics, hospitals, and pharmacies).
- Medical insurance (and what kind) individuals in that community use to access such services.

Such factors affect the settings and experiences that shape an audience's prototype expectations for healthcare.

After identifying the audience, creators of healthcare content can use methods such as surveys and questionnaires to collect context-related information from the intended audience. The resulting information can help in organizing individuals into groups (i.e., specific audiences for content) based on common experiences in healthcare contexts. After establishing such groups, content creators should ask a number of members from a group to participate in more direct data collection.

For these more direct activities, content creators could meet with individuals and conduct interviews, focus groups, or a mix of the two in order to collect richer information on healthcare experiences and expectations. Through such direct interactions, content creators can better identify that group's prototype expectations for healthcare activities. Per which method to use when collecting such information, each offers certain benefits:

- *Interviews* allow one to collect rich information on the opinions and perceptions of specific individuals, but this data reflects only one perspective.
- *Focus groups* allow one to collect information on a group's perspective through interactive group dynamics where individuals can comment on each other's statements and provide a more communal perspective on group perceptions. These dynamics, however, can inhibit some individuals from participating or affect the honesty of responses due to social concerns.
- *Mixed interviews and focus groups* allow one to collect both individual opinions and group perspectives, but they also often take more time to cordate data collection activities.

The number of interviews and focus groups to use depends on the time and resources (e.g., funding) available for such activities. Gathering as many perspectives as possible, however, is central to identifying patterns in how the population conceives of topics (Melonçon, 2017; St.Amant, 2017 & 2019a&b).

For this process, each method of data collection would involve the same questions asked in a certain order. Such an approach helps audience members conceptualize

- The prototypes of place they associate with a particular healthcare activity.
- The object prototypes they associate with the healthcare activity performed in that location.

Achieving this objective involves structuring and ordering interview/focus groups questions as follows:

Question 1: When do you do X (the process the writer wishes to document)?

Example: "When do you check your blood pressure?"

This initial question on time creates a context that helps audience members better conceptualize the prototypes of place associated with healthcare processes. If the initial question asked individuals "Where" they engage in healthcare activities, those persons might conceptualize an idealized situation for where they think they should go to receive care vs. the actual locations they visit. As a result, individuals might describe their prototype associations with an idealized vs. actual situation. Asking the "When" question thus prompts individuals to consider the time when they actually perform an activity and then access a more accurate prototype of place associated with a healthcare activity.

Question 2: Where do you do X (perform the healthcare activity) at Y (time activity takes place)?

Example: "Where do you check your blood pressure first thing in the morning?"

The first question primes individuals to thinking about timing ("When?"). This second question then asks individuals to identify the location where they perform a given healthcare activity at that time. This process allows individuals to access their prototype of place for the actual vs. idealize location where they perform that process.

Question 3: Can you describe X (location where care activity occurs) at Y (time of activity)? What is there? Who is there?

Example: Can you describe your kitchen at the start of the day? What is there? Who is there?

This third question helps individuals provide information on the features they associate with (and use to identify) the prototype of place expectations for a healthcare activity. As individuals respond, content creators/researchers need to ask them to describe the objects and persons in the area. Doing so helps identify the object prototypes respondents use to identify such items in that setting.

Such questioning involves identifying object prototypes within prototypes of place. These questions, therefore, need to be ordered in a way that helps identify the features associated with each kind of prototype. For example, if a respondent notes, "I go to the emergency room and there's a check-in counter and a lobby with chairs." the content creator/researcher should ask, "Can you describe the check-in counter for me?' and "Can you describe or draw me a picture of what the chairs look like and how they are arranged in that setting?" as well as "Can you do a sketch of how the check-in area is laid out? Where is the check-in counter? Where are the chairs and how are they arranged?" Such questioning helps create a more complete understanding of:

- The prototype of place individuals use to identify the location.
- The object prototypes used to identify items associated with identifying that location.

The resulting answers can provide insights into how an audience conceptualizes the process for which one will create informational or instructional content.

Question 4: Can you describe how you do X (process performed) in that place at that time?

Example: Can you describe how you take your blood pressure in your kitchen at the start of the day?

The question prompts individuals to describe how a particular process is performed, by whom, and using what items. Each aspect is central to understanding the mental models audiences rely on to understand and use content in order to achieve healthcare objectives.

Each step in this process has its own mental model that guides expectations of what an activity entails. The better one understands such nuances, the more effectively one can create content that addresses audience expectations in terms of health literacy factors (i.e., comprehension and usability). For this reason, gaining a complete understanding of such dynamics involves asking the following questions as individuals describe each step in a process:

Question 5: Who does X (specific activity)? Can you describe Y (item used)? Can you describe the overall activity?

Example: Who puts on the blood pressure cuff? What does the blood pressure cuff look like? What do they use to put the blood pressure cuff on?

As each activity within a process can involve its own actions, actors (who performs the process), and items (materials used to perform the process). Creating effective content for healthcare processes thus involves understanding the mental models guiding expectations for these actions. Doing so involves identifying the prototype expectations for each step in a process. For this reason, content creators/researchers need to ask these specific questions for each action individuals mention as they describe a healthcare process. For example, if an individual says, "The nurse takes my blood pressure by putting a device on my arm and then measuring it." The follow-up questions would be:

- "How do you know that person is a nurse? Can you describe that person for me?"
- "The item the nurse puts on your arm, what does it look like and/or feel like; can you describe it to me?"
- "What does the nurse do after putting the blood pressure device on your arm? Can you describe that process for me?"

Each response provides information on the prototypes individuals associate with these activities and can help in creating associated content (e.g., text or visuals) that matches such expectations.

Question 6: What do you do after you are done doing X (process performed)?

Example: "What do you do after you finish checking your blood pressure?"

The actions individuals describe when recounting a process might not encapsulate all activities related to a healthcare task. Rather, there could be additional actions that need to occur after the specific care-related activity is complete – activities that are actually part of the overall healthcare process. For example, individuals might be expected to take their blood pressure themselves, but then need to enter their systolic/diastolic numbers in a chart to track this information or to check in (e.g., call, email, or text) with a health care provider. These activities are a part of the overall healthcare process, but individuals might not perceive them as such and not include them when describing that process. Accordingly, content creators/researchers need to ask both this final question and follow-up questions as needed (e.g., "Can you describe how you do X/this follow-up process? What do you use? Can you describe that item?").

Designing and Testing Understanding

After collecting data on a healthcare activity, content creators need to review that information to identify aspects of the mental models an audience associates with a healthcare process. While differences among individuals will occur, the review process should focus on:

- Noting similarities across as many audience members as possible
- Identifying characteristics the overall group associates with

  - Recognizing a context of care (location)
  - Conceptualizing a caregiving process – what is used by whom and how.

Such commonalities can help to develop an initial checklist of factors to address when creating healthcare content to address the health literacy needs of the related audience. Content creators would then use these checklists to create initial content for the related audience. Ideally, such an approach would result in content that addresses the health literacy expectations and needs of the associated audience (St.Amant, 2017 & 2019b).

Content creators should not consider this initial checklist a final product. Rather, they need to test it with members of the intended audience to determine if revisions are needed. This testing could involve using the checklist to create sample images or draft text that identifies the location where a healthcare activity occurs and recount the related process per the items used to administer that care and the persons who participate in this process. Members of the intended audience would then review this draft content and – via interviews or focus groups – note how effectively such draft materials address their healthcare literacy expectations per prototypes of place and object prototypes (e.g., "I recognize/ don't' recognize this location/person/item. That is not how, in my experiences, the process is performed.") This review helps determine if members of the intended audience can effectively identify a location, item, person, or part of a process as conveyed in that draft content. If audience members cannot do so, content creators need to ask follow-up questions to determine why audience members could not:

- Understand parts (or all) of that content
- Recognize locations, persons, or items as depicted in that draft content

During this review process, content creators also need to ask audience members for suggestions on how to revise problematic content – what to change, add to, or remove from draft items – in order to address the audience's health literacy expectations per prototype associations.

Content creators would use this feedback to revise their design checklist and related content (e.g., images or text) and then test these revised materials with different individuals from the intended audience. If confusion and miscommunications again occur, content creators would again:

- Collect associated audience comments and revision suggestions.
- Revise the design checklist and associated draft content created using that checklist.
- Test this newly revised version with different members of the same audience.

This process of test, revise, and test the revised version would continue until (ideally) the audience has no problems using content or (pragmatically) time and funding for a project runs out. At a minimum, at least one round of testing should occur to determine how effectively content creators have addressed health literacy factors that guide the ways an audience uses healthcare content (St.Amant, 2017 & 2019a).

Concluding Thoughts

Mental models guide much of what individuals do every day. In health literacy contexts, these models can influence how individuals use informational and instructional materials. The better content creators understand such factors, the more effectively they can design materials to meet the health literacy practices of an audience. By understanding how prototypes affect conceptions of medical care, creators of healthcare content can develop materials that address the expectations affecting the needs of different groups. By employing the process described here, content creators – including undergraduate writing instructors and their students – can identify key health literacies and create content that audiences can use to achieve different healthcare objectives.

References

Acharya, K. R. (2019). Improving the quality of health care through human-centered design: Contextualizing design of biotechnology implementation for better health care and patient safety. *Present Tense: A Journal of Rhetoric in Society*, 7(3), 1–9.

Agboka, G. Y. (2014). Decolonial methodologies: Social justice perspectives in intercultural technical communication research. *Journal of Technical Writing and Communication*, 44(3), 297–327

Aitchison, J. (1994). Bad birds and better birds: Prototype theory. In V. P. Clark, P. A. Eschholz, & A. F. Rosa (Eds.), *Language: Introductory readings*, 4th ed. (pp. 445–459). New York: St. Martins Press.

Eyal, N. (2014). *Hooked: How to build habit-forming products*. New York: Portfolio/Penguin Books.

health.gov. (2021). Health literacy in Healthy People 2030. https://health.gov/our-work/national-health-initiatives/healthy-people/healthy-people-2030/health-literacy-healthy-people-2030

Interaction Design Foundation. (n. d.). Usability. https://www.interaction-design.org/literature/topics/usability

Lindstrom, M. (2010). *Buyology: Truth and lies about why we buy*. New York: Broadway Books.

Melonçon, L. (2017). Patient experience design: Expanding usability methodologies for healthcare. *Communication Design Quarterly*, 5(2), 19–28.

Melonçon, L. (2016). Patient experience design: Technical communication's role in patient health information and education. *Intercom*, 62(2), 12–16. www.ccnsus.gov/library/stories/2018/10/snapshot-fast-growing-us-older-population.html

Rosch, E. (1978). Principles of categorization. In E. Rosch & B. L. Lloyd (Eds.), *Cognition and categorization* (pp. 27–48). Hillsdale, NJ: Lawrence Erlbaum.

Saru, E. H., & Wojan, P. (2020). Glocalization: Of health information: Considering design factors for mobile technologies in Malaysia. *Journal of Technical Writing and Communication*, 50(2), 187–206.

St.Amant, K. (2019a). The cultural context for communicating care. *Journal of Technical Writing and Communication*, 49(4), 367–382.

St.Amant, K. (2019b, May/June). Usability in contexts of care. *Intercom*, 66(3), 35–36.

St.Amant, K. (2018a, Nov.). Usable design – Giving users what they expect. *tcWorld*, 2018(4), 25–28.

St.Amant, K. (2018b). Reflexes, reactions, and usability: Examining how prototypes of place can enhance UXD practices. *Communication Design Quarterly*, 6(1), 45–53.

St.Amant, K. (2017). The cultural context of care in international communication design: A heuristic for addressing usability in international health and medical communication. *Communication Design Quarterly*, 5(2), 62–70.

St.Amant, K. (2015). Culture and the contextualization of care: A prototype-based approach to developing health and medical visuals for international audiences. *Communication Design Quarterly*, 3(2), 38–47.

Wolfe, J. M. (2007). *Guided search 4.0: Current progress with a model of visual search. Integrated models of cognitive systems*. New York, NY: Oxford University Press, 2007.

Wolfe, J. M. (1994). Guided search 2.0: A revised model of visual search. *Psychonomic Bulletin and Review*, 1(2), 202–238.

World Health Organization. (2022). Improving health literacy. https://www.who.int/activities/improving-health-literacy

INDEX

Note: **Bold** page numbers refer to tables and *italic* page numbers refer to figures.